THE JOURNAL OF

William Tully

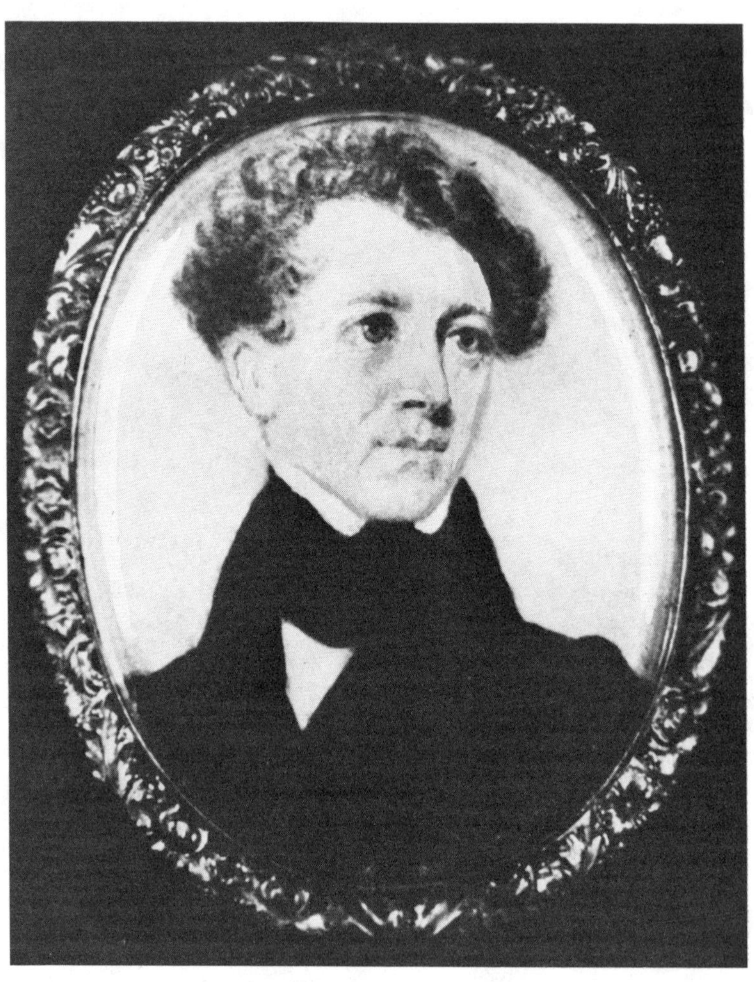

A miniature of the young William Tully painted by Thomas H. Parker in watercolor on ivory. *Yale University Art Gallery, Gift of Mrs. John Hill Morgan, The Leila A. and John Hill Morgan Collection.*

THE JOURNAL OF
William Tully

Medical Student at Dartmouth
1808 - 1809

OLIVER S. HAYWARD

ELIZABETH H. THOMSON

Editors

Foreword by
JOHN F. FULTON

NEW YORK 1977

SCIENCE HISTORY PUBLICATIONS

First published in 1977 by
Science History Publications
a division of
Neale Watson Academic Publications, Inc.
156 Fifth Avenue, New York 10010

William Tully's Journal is published
with the kind permission of the
Beinecke Rare Book and Manuscript Library,
Yale University Library.
Endpapers are taken from pages
8 and 9, 66 and 67, vol. III.

Library of Congress Cataloging in Publication Data
Tully, William, 1785–1859.
   The journal of William Tully, medical student
at Dartmouth, 1808–1809.

   1. Pharmacology.   2. Pharmacologists—Connecti-
cut—Biography.   3. Tully, William, 1785–1859.
RM88.T84   1977   615'.092'4 [B]   77–13727
ISBN 0–88202–175–3

Composed, printed and bound at the Haddon Craftsmen,
Scranton, Pennsylvania, U.S.A.
Designer: Ernst Reichl

PREFACE

When John F. Fulton, Sterling Professor of the History of Medicine at the Yale University School of Medicine, spent a year at New London, New Hampshire recovering from a serious illness (1957–1958), his physician was a local practitioner, Oliver S. Hayward. During their almost daily contacts an element of the curative regimen was frequent discussion of a man they mutually admired—the justly renowned surgeon-physician Nathan Smith. Since Dr. Hayward's career paralleled Smith's to some degree— he was also a Harvard Medical School graduate and a country doctor serving the same area in which Smith had practiced, he felt a particular affinity to Smith, had gathered some material about him, and was eager to attempt a full-length study, long needed, of the scope of his contributions to medical practice and medical education.

In this formidable ambition Dr. Fulton encouraged Oliver Hayward with the ultimate result that he joined him as a Principal Investigator in an application for a supportive grant from the National Institutes of Health. In 1959 they were awarded a three-year grant for a definitive study of Nathan Smith which awaits only final revision and publication. Miss Margaret Abbott, a graduate of Simmons College well trained in research, fortunately lived in New London and became research assistant and secretary to the project. Dr. Hayward forthwith began an intensive search for original materials and other information about the practice of Nathan Smith, his patients, his students, his friends and associates, and his role as one of the pre-eminent surgeons and medical educators in New England in the early nineteenth century.

In the course of his investigation Dr. Hayward made a valuable find at Yale University—the journal of William Tully (B.A. Yale 1806), one of Smith's most illustrious pupils, which he kept while studying under him during 1808–1809 at Dartmouth where Smith had founded, singlehanded, the fourth school of medicine in the country (1797). The Journal was the gift of the Misses Tully, his two surviving daughters, in 1896.

With painstaking care Miss Abbott transcribed Tully's often difficult handwriting while Dr. Hayward investigated Tully's life and career for the Essay which follows. Meanwhile he drew not only Dr. Fulton into the enterprise, persuading him to write a Foreword, but other members and associates of his Department of the History of Medicine as well. Dr. Whitfield J. Bell, Jr., then Associate Editor of the Franklin Papers at Yale, had for so long been a steady contributor to medical history that he naturally was welcomed as a consultant and adviser in Department activities. Dr. Hayward was grateful for his considerable help with the introductory essay and in the annotation of the Journal. Miss Madeline E. Stanton, Librarian of the Historical Library in the Yale Medical Library, gave generously of her time and her special knowledge of the resources available. I was invited to cast an editorial eye over the manuscript as a whole, to modernize the punctuation by omitting the excessive number of commas and capitals which stood in the way of the modern reader's enjoyment of the text, and to assume responsibility for the final preparation for publication. Miss Marjorie G. Wynne, presently Edwin J. Beinecke Research Librarian at the Beinecke Rare Book and Manuscript Library, was most helpful in regard to the use of the Journal and in securing permission to publish the manuscript.

In 1959 and 1960, however, a publisher who did not require a sizeable subvention was not to be found. Shortly after Dr. Fulton's death in May 1960 Oliver Hayward went to the National Institutes of Health to work in cancer chemotherapy and thence into clinical research and therapy among heroin addicts. Both jobs were too demanding to be combined with historical research. Tully's Journal meantime has waited in the Department files for

increased interest in original material of this nature and for a
publisher with courage and appreciation of its value in the widen-
ing study of sources which have relevance to our interpretation of
medical history today.

ELIZABETH H. THOMSON

Department of the History of Science and Medicine
Yale University School of Medicine
August 1977

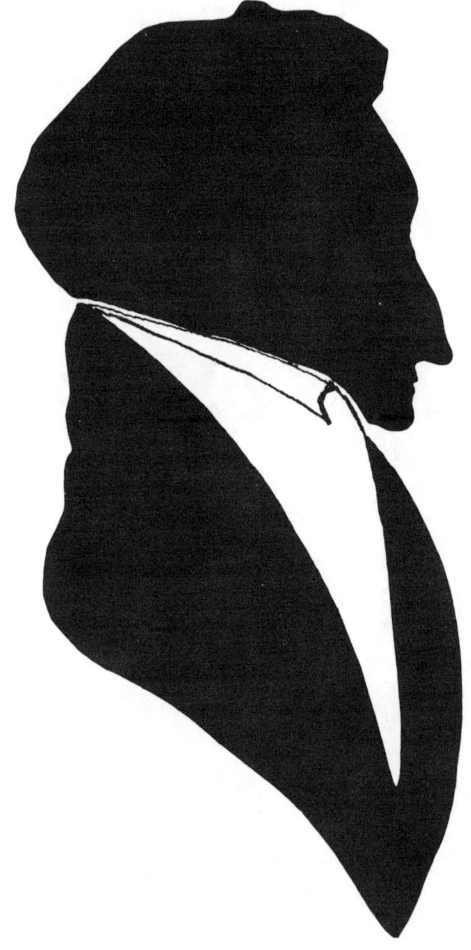

A silhouette of Dr. Nathan Smith (1762–1828). Artist unknown. *Courtesy of the Dartmouth College Library.*

FOREWORD

On the 15th of September 1808 William Tully, a Yale graduate of the Class of 1806, set forth from his home in Saybrook, Connecticut, for Hanover, New Hampshire, where he was to enter the Dartmouth Medical School. During the preceding year he had been studying medicine apprenticed to an established physician, as was the custom of the times, his preceptor being the eminent Dr. Mason F. Cogswell of Hartford. His training in the profession of his choice had therefore already begun—and very satisfactorily for him. The next stage in his education was to start under circumstances considerably less favorable from his point of view.

Tully kept an almost day-by-day diary of his three months in Hanover. Since he was a bright, intelligent young man with keen powers of observation, his comments on his fellow travellers and the towns and people seen during the four-day journey by stagecoach, his impressions of Hanover, its taverns, its people, and its college—buildings, faculty, and students—are of considerable interest. To anyone concerned with general or social history of the nineteenth century his comments on the customs of the time, his comparisons between the more opulent life in Connecticut and the rural life of Hanover not yet far removed from frontier days are a rich source of information. But Tully's diary is most important for its mirror of Nathan Smith, the country doctor who served five medical schools and who was one of the outstanding physicians and educators of his day. His reputation has gathered luster through the years as time has afforded the perspective necessary to bring out his true stature. An intimate view of him as both teacher and physician through the eyes of a critical student is therefore of particular significance.

Tully's frequent comparisons between Dartmouth and Yale in respect to faculty, equipment, dress, etc. will amuse any member of the 'Ivy League' communities except possibly those connected with Dartmouth. But his journal will appeal to a far larger audience, for lively opinions, indignantly expressed, are often entertaining even if the author reveals himself as a provincial, opinionated, and pious young man not exactly devoid of what James Russell Lowell called "the elbowing self-conceit of youth." He had no obvious sense of humor, but he did show a certain honesty in retracting some of his first unfavorable opinions so positively stated, and occasionally he exhibited earnest efforts to be broadminded and philosophical. Fortunately for him, he discovered two or three other Yale men among his classmates; thus was life made more tolerable.

Tully was fairly well impressed with Dr. Smith though he commented on the fact that as he waited for Smith to read his letters of introduction, the professor made no effort to introduce him to the three ladies of the family who were sewing in the room. Nor was he introduced later when he was cordially invited to join the family at dinner. The conversation during the meal was recorded in detail. Dr. Smith was interested in the plans for a medical school at Yale but thought the College authorities would do well to avoid the affiliation with the State Medical Society that they were contemplating. He felt state legislatures should help to provide buildings and apparatus, but "the emolument to the Teacher ought to come from the Pupils. . . ." Harvard University was named as an example of the ruinous effects of salaries being provided for the Faculty by the Institution, since the professors had been making no improvements in their lectures since about the year 1750. He considered Yale "as now having the preëminence of every College in the Country, and as in the fairest way to preserve it" if President Dwight lived long enough to put his excellent plans for improvement into execution.

Such opinions must have been gratifying to the homesick Yale graduate who was also pleased to hear his most admired Yale professor, Benjamin Silliman, called "the first Chemist in New England."

Then came the day of the first medical lecture. Tully arrived early and observed his fellow students closely. "Such a motley colection I am sure I never set my eyes on before." Their clothes "were, in general, so ludicrously put on that I hardly dared to trust myself with a second view." He did find, however, that the appearance and deportment of several denoted the complete gentleman and he went on to say: "On reviewing the company they did not appear half as bad as at first, and I perceived at last that much of my disgust arose from the total want of uniformity among them. I felt forcibly the propriety of establishing a uniform for all members of literary Institutions, and I began to be conscious that much of the applause that the Students of Yale-College have gained for their appearance has been owing to a similarity of dress and behavior which they generally fall into by the end of the first term Freshman-Year."

Dr. Smith slipped into the room unnoticed by the students. Tully wrote that he had been expecting some of Professor Silliman's majesty and grace and felt a kind of disgust from his disappointment. He continued: "His Introductory address was altogether extemporaneous and couched in the most colloquial phrases. It was pithy, however, and in spite of its want of elegance, I could not but like it tolerably well. By this time I had got past being disappointed at anything that I should meet in Hanover, and I made up my mind to be attentive to the matter only and not the manner of what my Instructor and fellow Students should say. As I had just got into this frame of mind, the embarrassment of the Doctor's first address was over, and the man of true erudition, and the master of his Profession was manifest."

This opinion was reinforced during the three months he studied under Smith. On December 28th, six days before he left Hanover, he set down his final impressions of Dartmouth, its faculty and methods of instruction, closing his remarks with "Of Dr. Smith's School, which is connected with the College, I cannot speak too highly. . . ."

Back in Saybrook, on the 4th of January, William Tully made

the last entry in this diary so rich in human interest. Only a few years later Nathan Smith was to be the big drawing card on the faculty of the Medical Institution of Yale College when it opened its doors in the autumn of 1813. This man, whom Alan Gregg, himself a great medical educator, happily described as "the Johnny Appleseed of American medical education," was to leave an indelible mark also on the Yale Medical School and on other schools still to come. His one-time student, William Tully, who served on its faculty from 1829 to 1842, was likewise to leave his mark, for he developed into a colorful individualist, as any reader of his diary might have forecast. He became an outstanding teacher, author, and physician who earned a secure place for himself in the history of nineteenth century medicine.

JOHN F. FULTON, M.D.

New London, New Hampshire
25 August 1958

ESSAY ON WILLIAM TULLY

Oliver S. Hayward, M.D.

William Tully, Bachelor of Arts of Yale, 1806, was angry. Soberly dressed, as all Yale graduates and serious students of medicine should be, he was sitting in the dark, low-hung Dartmouth College chapel, a guest at Quarter-Day Public Speaking. His work in the medical classes had not been too confining, he was only two years out of college, and he had thought by attending the public speaking to learn how things were done in this young institution at Hanover. The chapel had filled rapidly with roughly dressed, boisterous countrymen, who were Dartmouth students. Dr. John Smith, professor of languages and an ordained clergyman, had introduced the unprepossessing junior who was now reciting. It was no classical dissertation, but a parody of Peter Pindar directed against medical students. As the boy spoke, now with rushing earnestness, now with ill-concealed mirth, he grinned at the medical students' discomfiture. This was one way to pay them back for their patronizing or disdainful manner to undergraduates! The reaction was hardly in the best of taste, but most listeners would have let it pass. But William Tully reddened, grew angry with this "dirty little Scoundrel," and, returning hastily to his room, wrote a protest calculated, as he thought, to teach these New Hampshire boors better manners. This he intended to have published in the *Hanover Gazette*.

What, one asks, was so humorless, censorious, and complacent a young man doing in Hanover at all? He had come there to study medicine under Dr. Nathan Smith, Professor of Medicine in the College. During ten years of teaching all the medical courses at Dartmouth, Nathan Smith had established a reputation as a master of medicine, original in thought and fearless in accepting or rejecting the authority of the old and famous. Smith's own fame had spread beyond New Hampshire, and even a Connecticut man like Tully might feel that medicine was better taught at Hanover than in New York, Philadelphia, or Boston. As for Connecticut, medicine was not taught there at all, except by practising physicians to their apprentices.

William Tully's first American ancestors—a widow and two young children—came from England to Saybrook, Connecticut, in 1646 or 1647. The widow's son, John, had inherited property in England, but when the time came to claim it he discovered to his dismay that the parchment deeds had been cut up for patterns for embroidery. Systematically, however, he reassembled the pieces; the Widow Tully sewed them together; and, carrying this patchwork of English law and New England needlework, John Tully successfully pressed his claims through the courts and returned to Saybrook, where he married in 1671. With a better-than-average education and no taste for farming, John Tully sold his lands and became a schoolmaster, teaching arithmetic, navigation, and astronomy. Each year after 1681 he furnished the astronomical calculations for a series of almanacs printed at Boston. He was town clerk for many years, and he increased his income by acting as a scrivener. His learning and unusual common sense even won him the reputation of a wizard or conjuror among his ignorant and superstitious neighbors. An instance of this was preserved by a family chronicler: a person whose child had been lost in the woods on Long Island applied to Tully several months later; on learning that no search had been made in an Indian village near where the child was last seen, Tully directed the father to inquire there, which he did, and found his child safe.

For more than a century before our William Tully's birth in 1785, his family had produced a succession of intelligent, substantial, but undistinguished citizens of Saybrook. John Tully's son William was a tanner and shoemaker, and the diarist's father was Colonel William Tully of the Connecticut militia. Three

xiv

Tullys served long periods as town clerks; one was a member of the legislature; all were active church members. Tully's uncle and cousin were captains of the militia.

Dr. William Tully was born on 18 November 1785, in the house his grandfather had built at Saybrook Point. This house still stands on North Cove Road, near the southern end of the Cove, overlooking the Connecticut River. From its windows one could look across the marshes to the village of Saybrook, with the low-lying hills beyond, and out over Long Island Sound. Little is known of Tully's boyhood, but it must have been a pleasant one, for throughout his life he retained a deep affection for his birthplace and his early friends there. He attended the district school and was tutored by the Rev. Mr. Frederick W. Hotchkiss, minister of the First Congregational Church in Saybrook and a Yale graduate. This preparation, though doubtless superior to what was available to most New England boys, was, Tully confessed later, "exceedingly defective, especially in arithmetic."

He entered Yale in 1802 at the age of 17. He made some special friends (with one of them, Henry Fish, he went to Hanover), he was elected to the Linonian Society, and he became an honorary member of Phi Beta Kappa. Though only a small town, New Haven seemed a cosmopolitan metropolis compared to Saybrook; and the college gave young Tully standards of intellectual and social comparison which he carried through life. Northampton, Massachusetts, was important to him because it was the birthplace of President Dwight of Yale; and a New Hampshire town was not wholly negligible if some Yale alumnus was living there. Tully quoted with approval his tutor Hotchkiss's remark that spending four years under Dwight and the faculty at Yale spoiled a man for liking anyone else.

Somewhere, possibly while at college, Tully learned to cut silhouettes, and is said to have made portraits of 27 members of his class, including himself, which he thought "a poor likeness." He was graduated in 1806, standing so high in his class that he would have been valedictorian, he believed, but for the lack in his early arithmetical training. A miniature painted of him about this time shows a handsome, sensitive, delicately featured young man, perhaps a little apprehensive of the world he was entering.

It was a world of gusty political storms. When William Tully was graduated at Yale, Thomas Jefferson was President; and to Jefferson and his followers New England Federalists applied the most opprobrious epithet they knew—Democratic Republicans. Jeffersonian doctrine and policy, which seemed to take a complaisant view of the excesses of popular control in the French Revolution, deeply offended New England's cherished political and social convictions; while New England's trade was caught up in the great struggle then waging between England and France. Between 1807 and 1808 American exports dropped from $108 million to $22.5 million.

At the same time Congregational ministers in scores of New England meetinghouses flayed Jefferson as anti-Christ and his religion as atheism. President Dwight of Yale was one of the most articulate and influential defenders of the old religion against the rationalism of the lingering eighteenth century. His students, men like Tully, though they were not devoutly Christian, were his strong supporters. To William Tully, from a comfortable home and an assured position in Saybrook, radicalism of any kind was shocking and foolish, if not worse. He disliked "bustles of all kinds, and especially Political ones." He had little sympathy with the *"Sovereign People,"* and said contemptuously of one democratic politician that the best way to get rid of him "would be to give him an office, which, I am sure, would puff him up so much, that he would ultimately burst." So much a part of him was his conservative attitude that, though otherwise a good judge of character, Tully had a closed mind on religion and politics; and he could accept only with great reluctance the bona fides of anyone who was not both a good Congregationalist and a good Federalist. In his latter years his monologues and tirades on religion and politics were notorious for their vehemence.

The first winter after his graduation from Yale Tully spent as a schoolmaster at the Oyster River District School in Saybrook. In the spring of 1807, however, he went to Hartford to begin the study of medicine under Dr. Mason F. Cogswell. "In the Doctor,"

xvi

Tully wrote appreciatively, "extensive Science, correct literary taste, and the utmost suavity and elegance of manners are happily combined"; and he received "nothing but kindness and the most flattering attention" from his master during the year and a half he worked with him.

Medical training took many forms in the eighteenth century and early nineteenth. At one extreme medicine was practiced by persons, often ministers, who had had no medical education at all, but were the only educated men in the community, so that their neighbors called on them for help in time of illness. At the other extreme were the physicians, still few but growing in number, who had been trained in the famous medical schools of Europe. But the great majority of young men wishing to become doctors spent several years with a practicing physician and then, provided with a certificate and a measure of self-confidence, began to practice. If things did not go too badly, they continued to practice, acquired experience and skill, and in time became useful and valuable. Nathan Smith, for example, under whom Tully studied at Hanover, first practiced successfully at Cornish, New Hampshire, for three years with no other preparation than a term as apprentice under Dr. Josiah Goodhue.

But Nathan Smith had left Cornish to study at the Harvard Medical School, and after Harvard he had spent a year in London and Edinburgh before beginning to teach and practice at Hanover. Medical education, as Smith's career illustrates, was in transition. With the establishment of medical schools throughout the country, it became easier for students to take formal instruction in addition to the practical experience of apprenticeship. Soon attendance at a medical school, whether good or bad, became the prevailing pattern. Even then, however, there was no graded curriculum; a student heard the same lectures a second or a third year, if he stayed that long; he might or might not obtain a degree; and, if he did, the degree might be that of doctor of medicine or of bachelor of medicine. Even with a degree, since there were no systems of general state licensing, he was legally in no better position than plausible rascals who sold cancer cures to the gullible and the desperate. Even William Tully, for example, never had an M.B. degree, and he did not receive an M.D. (from Yale!) until after he had been in practice for ten years. Rather surprisingly Dartmouth College has no record that Tully ever attended its Medical School.

For all its evident deficiencies, the apprentice system of medical education was not all bad. Many able physicians came out of it. At its best it provided an intelligent, observant, hard-working youth with incomparable practical experience. Its irreparable defect was that it gave a student so little of the theoretical foundation of medical knowledge. For that one must go to the schools; and that is why, in the fall of 1808, William Tully left Dr. Cogswell and travelled to Hanover and Nathan Smith.

Going to Hanover was not altogether an agreeable experience for Tully, even though it was a part of his professional preparation. Hanover had little to remind him of Saybrook and New Haven, and Dartmouth was not Yale. He looked in vain for a house as friendly and attractive as the one he left, for a church as beautiful and soaring as the new one in Hartford, for the pleasant mixture of intellectual and social talk he had known in the Linonian Society. In Hanover he was a stranger; his journal records his disgust with the dirty inns, his awkwardness in the presence of the "natives," whose manners were so different from his own. He seriously considered returning home at once; but his anger and his sense of superiority to all things "New-Hantonian" and Dartmuthiensis were stronger than his loneliness. He even set down Nathan Smith at first as another countryman with the rest, although he allowed that Smith was like "a Connecticut farmer," which was, of course, considerably higher than one from New Hampshire or Massachusetts.

Nathan Smith was a Yankee of the best kind. He had been a farmer and a schoolmaster when, deciding to study medicine at the age of 24, he became an apprentice to Dr. Goodhue, of Chester, Vermont, a skillful surgeon and competent medical teacher, who was later President of the Berkshire Medical School. For a while Smith practiced at Cornish, New Hampshire, and then, wanting more formal training, took a year off to study at Harvard under Dr. John Warren and Dr. Benjamin Waterhouse, the latter a nephew of the celebrated John Fothergill of London and a graduate of Leyden. Smith received the degree of M.B. in 1790. Six more years of country practice followed. Then, somehow, he financed a year of study in London and Edinburgh in 1796–1797, crowning his studies by election as a corresponding member of the Medical Society of London. This year of foreign study Smith undertook with the idea of founding a medical school at Hanover when he returned; and he had received the approval and encouragement of the Dartmouth trustees (but no financial aid). He returned home in 1797 and, with Lyman Spalding, a former student, as instructor in chemistry, he opened his school and began to lecture.

In the ten years that the Dartmouth Medical School had been open, it had graduated several young men who were already well known in New England. Smith's first graduate, Joseph Gallup, had been the second man to vaccinate with kine pox in Vermont; he was to found the Vermont Medical Society and become professor and President of the Vermont Medical Academy in Castleton. Amos Twitchell, a graduate of 1805, was practicing in Keene, New Hampshire, with such success that, it is said, during his career he was offered professorships in twelve different medical colleges. And Lyman Spalding, who had studied under Smith at Cornish and helped him at the opening of the School, returned to Hanover as a student in 1808; he was later chairman of the commission which supervised the compilation of the first American pharmacopoeia in 1820.

Tully knew these things about his teacher. What he was not prepared for was Smith's forthright, rustic manner; his extemporaneous lectures, his colloquial speech were so unlike the "majesty and grace" of Professor Silliman at Yale that Tully was embarrassed for him. But the young man could not indulge his attitudes of superiority long. Smith's evident mastery of his subject, the vigor and honesty of his mind, his precise, lucid, and pithy statements carried all before them. Within six weeks young Tully had almost forgotten Yale and was writing that the students "admired and revered" Smith "more and more as we know him better."

As a practicing physician as well as a professor, Smith could offer his students opportunities to witness his treatments, especially surgical operations. Most patients were operated on in their own homes; it was not until 1809 that Smith provided for demonstrations of surgical operations before his classes by erecting a new "Medical House" complete with an ingenious trolley by which the patients might be wheeled in and out. One of his students has described how, when Smith sent word that he was going to operate in the country, the young men would saddle up and ride out with their professor. "Almost all our conversation took the form of clinical lectures and was at all times interesting and instructive. . . . Occasionally in our long rides, when we were kept from home for a night, Dr. Smith would retire to his room and write a chapter or a few pages for his forthcoming work. . . ." Tully, however, never accompanied Smith and his classmates on such visits. The reason he gives in his Journal—that they took him away from his books, which were more valuable—does not seem honest. A more likely reason, supported by the tone of the Journal and Tully's subsequent career, is that he could not bear the sight of surgery without anesthesia.

Tully's Journal provides some interesting pictures of medical students' life at Hanover early in the nineteenth century. He was one of four young men who met twice weekly to review their work together. Not content only to go over their notes, each occasionally wrote some composition on a medical subject, which he read for the criticism of the others. Doubtless other groups of friends met similarly during the fall and winter nights.

More interesting and significant is what Tully has to say of a society of medical students known as The High Court. It began merely as a social group, "and to tell the truth, all the Good Fellows, either among the Medical-Students or the Dartmouth Graduates belonged to it," Tully wrote. Membership was by invitation, many fewer than half the medical students were in it, but they were the better educated, the more mannerly, the gentlemen and good fellows. The students with whom Smith associated personally outside of class were apt to be members of the High Court, not because of that, of course, but because they were better educated and had better manners. In addition, the High

Court had a badge, which its members displayed prominently. For all these reasons, the majority of the medical students deeply resented the society. The division in the Medical School thus created was aggravated, as Tully relates, by the publication of a catalogue of students' names. What the High Court members and their sympathizers like Tully opposed in the idea of a catalogue was having their names appear on the same list with ill-educated New Hampshire clodhoppers.

Tully returned to Hanover for a second course of lectures in 1809. Then or earlier he determined to make materia medica his special study. In January 1810 he was studying with Dr. Samuel Carter at Saybrook; and in March, having returned to New Haven, he entered the office of Dr. Eli Ives, Yale's Professor of Materia Medica, giving special attention to botany. The Connecticut Medical Society gave him a license to practice in October 1810. He returned to Saybrook that winter, however, and taught school. Then in May 1811 he settled at Enfield, Connecticut, and two years later married Mary Potter, daughter of the Reverend Mr. Elam O. Potter of Enfield.

Tully's youth was now over. He moved about so much, practicing in so many communities, that one biographer has called him "the peregrinating Dr. William Tully." He was at Enfield from 1811 to 1813; at Milford for eight months; then back to Enfield. In 1815 he moved to Cromwell, and in 1818 to Middletown. In 1822 he moved to East Hartford; in 1824 he was appointed President and Professor of the Theory and Practice of Medical Jurisprudence in the Vermont Academy of Medicine at Castleton. In 1826 he moved to Albany, New York, and in 1829 Yale invited him to take the chair of Materia Medica and Therapeutics just vacated by the death of his old teacher, Eli Ives. After much debate he accepted the appointment though he is said to have resigned regularly once a year thereafter. He was a popular teacher, and his students repeatedly manifested their enthusiasm for his lectures. Meanwhile he had begun to write. His first article was "On the Ergot of Rye" in the *American Journal of Science* in 1820. Other articles followed; in 1823, with Dr. Thomas Miner, he published "Essays on Fevers." He prepared a catalogue of wild plants and ferns growing in the vicinity of New Haven, and in 1857 a massive compendium appeared in two volumes, entitled, *Materia Medica, or, Pharmacology and Therapeutics*. This was to have been the first section of an eighteen-volume work.

Even now William Tully's peregrinations were not at an end. Because of strained relations with his colleagues at Yale, he resigned his post in 1842, though he continued to live in New Haven until 1851, when he moved to Springfield, Massachusetts. There he died on 28 February 1859; he was buried in Grove Street Cemetery, New Haven.

Prof. Henry Bronson, who knew him well and succeeeded him at Yale, gave a detailed appraisal of the man in the *Boston Medical and Surgical Journal* (1861, *65*, 54–60):

Dr. Tully was doubtless the most learned and thoroughly scientific physician in New England. If his equal may be found anywhere, I am ignorant of the fact. He had a large and costly library, and was a diligent and methodical student through life. His knowledge of botany was extensive and very accurate. Chemistry, particularly organic and pharmaceutical chemistry, he understood probably better than any one in this country. He was acquainted with physiology, and was familiar with the literature of these branches of his profession which he did not practise. Indeed, his studies took a wide range. He knew Latin and Greek well, at least so far as these languages are employed in natural science. And all his knowledge was singularly minute and exact. He assisted Dr. [Noah] Webster and Prof. Goodrich in the scientific department of their dictionary, furnishing the definitions of the terms of Anatomy, Physiology, Medicine, Botany, and some other branches of natural history. . . .

Tully was a tall man and handsome, with a commanding presence. Having a forceful personality and some novel and bold views which he pronounced with great vigor, he was a favorite among the students who always admire those of their teachers who for one reason or another stand out from their fellows, and who are fearless in offering criticism, whether of men or of books. Some students went so far as to ape some of his peculiarities of manner or imitate the stentorian tones of his voice. Nevertheless, Tully's private students were thoroughly trained and many became distinguished in their own right, for despite his strong prejudices and a somewhat quixotic temperament, he was a highly intelligent and discriminating physician. Bronson appraised him thus:

> He investigated his cases thoroughly, usually arrived at a correct diagnosis, drew inferences cautiously, and grounded his opinions on the facts before him. His unrivalled knowledge of materia medica, particularly indigenous materia medica, and his familiarity with all the new remedies, especially the new organic compounds, gave him a great advantage in prescription. His resources in a difficult case were, as far as I know, unparalleled. He was somewhat famous for the treatment of obstinate chronic cases—cases that had worn out the patience of others. . . . And he not unfrequently succeeded in curing diseases which had defied the skill of the ablest and best practitioners. . .

Perhaps the secret of his success lay in the fact that he was fond of what Bronson calls 'heroic' medicines and treatment, scorning some of the mild remedies in common use and the customary blood-letting, cathartics, antimony, etc. He used alcohol, morphine, quinine, strychnine, arsenic, and the like, and he used these with the confidence of a man who has faith in himself and his own judgments. Once he had formed his opinions, he was unyielding, even headstrong, as forceful men are apt to be, and he brooked no interference with his orders on the part of nurses, patients, or their families and friends. This did not always enhance his popularity as a physician, but he was nevertheless warmly admired for his courage and his integrity. A biographer wrote that "no act of meanness or low malice tarnishes his fair name," adding that his relationships with other practitioners were always highly honorable.

Tully loved to join with medical friends in conversation but the result was usually more of a monologue than a dialogue! However, the range of his curiosity and his enthusiasm made him a stimulating companion, and his knowledge of words which he "loved, seemingly, for their own sake," no doubt accounted for his close friendship with Noah Webster, the great Connecticut lexicographer.

In his Journal there is already much of the man he was to become—a man quick to make judgments, exuberant when his admiration had been won, brilliant, strong-minded, contentious—a man of wide interests which he pursued with intensity and intelligence. He showed little wit or humor then or later, but his Journal is a lively, human document of more than ordinary interest and flavor which reveals the first flowering of a personality which was to wield a strong influence on medical education and also on the progress of medicine itself in nineteenth century New England.

William Tully's
Journal
1808 - 1809

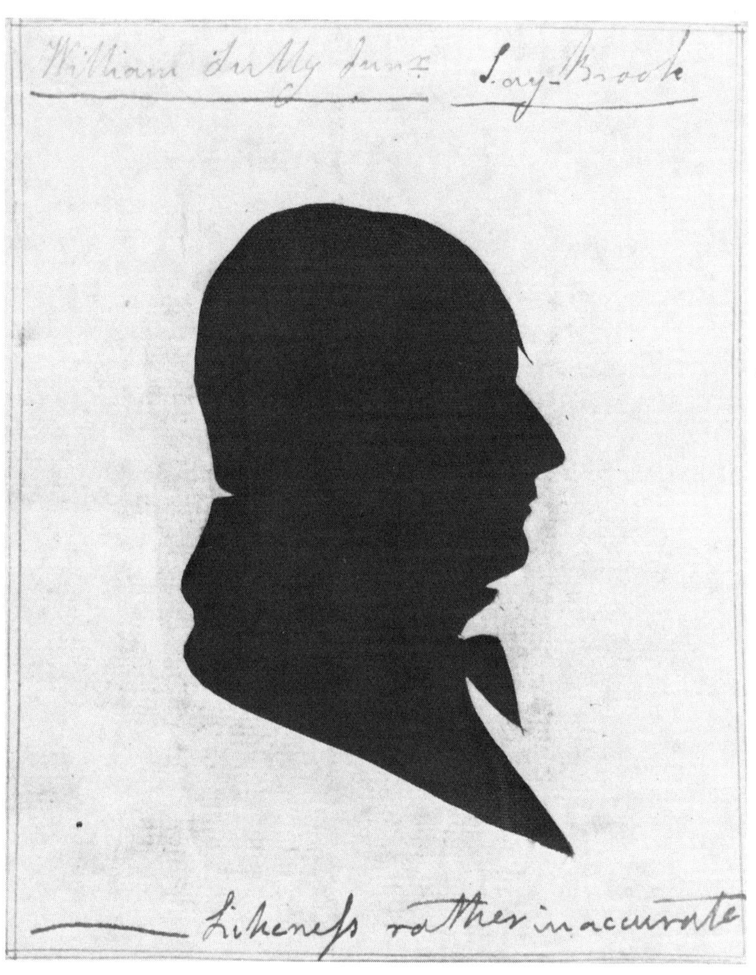

A silhouette of William Tully done by Tully himself. From his "Profiles of the Class that was admitted into Yale College September A.D. 1802." *Yale University Archives, Yale University Library.*

IT IS an old Proverb that a man is known by the company he keeps.

It must, therefore, be a source of much satisfaction to be able to look back, after a lapse of years, and ascertain from actually written record that one has no cause to blush for his associates, and consequently for his actions and habits. When, too, one is accustomed to note precisely the manner in which his time is passed, the desire of a pleasing retrospect, at the year's end, will be a powerfull motive to a becoming circumspection in all his conduct, and a knowledge that his transactions will stare him in the face as often as he looks into his Journal will prove a strong stimulus to an irreproachable life.

From these considerations, and many others, I purpose tomorrow to commence something of this kind, as I shall then leave Say-Brook, and my natural guardians, for a long absence; and God grant that my conduct may be such that an account of it will give all my friends pleasure.

Friday 16th.

Departed from the place of my nativity and the scenes of my childhood but with sensations far different from what most people feel on a like occasion. Were all precisely in my circumstances, however, all would, in my view, have felt as I did. I had never had intimates in Say-Brook, and but few natural relations. Of these I had just taken leave, after having made them a long visit. I expected to hear often from them, and what should remain then to prevent me from going whither my interest should lead. Abstracted local attachments never existed in my heart.

My companions, as far as Hartford, were my Father, Mr. William Lynde, a wealthy and sensible farmer, Mr. Nathaniel Clarke, a man of much humour and shrewdness, and my excentric cousin John Ingraham, all of Say-Brook. The three first were going to act as Grand-Jurors to the Federal-Court, just about to be in session; Ingraham for a visit to his father in Enfield; and I intended to take the stage the next Thursday for Dartmouth-College for the purpose of finishing my medical-education under Professor N. Smith. From the time that we should arrive in our Metropolis to the time of my departure from it I promised myself abundant leisure to visit old friends.

We all, about noon, embarked from Captain Dickinson's Wharf in an elegant little Vineyard boat with a light breeze southeasterly, and sailed moderately up the Connecticut. The season was charming for such an expedition and had not I recently had several unpleasant passages under almost similar circumstances, I should have anticipated much pleasure from the cruise. Mr. Lynde, however, by his entertaining remarks, Mr. Clarke with his wit, and Cousin Jack with his *outré* manner of doing and saying every thing completely beguiled me of the tediousness of the way, and we found ourselves at Knowles'-Landing about sunset. We made but a short stop, for our prospect for proceeding was favourable and we hoped to reach Hartford in the evening; and so we did, but at a much later hour than we calculated. Indeed, I believe it was after midnight before we landed, and probably another hour before we got well in bed. We tarried at Knox's near the waterside in the northern part of the town.

Saturday 17th.

Awoke as early as usual, notwithstanding my late hours the preceeding night.

The morning was cloudy and occasionally there fell light showers of rain.

I made it my first business to see Doctor Cogswell[1] and his amiable family.

In his house, and under his immediate instruction and guardianship, I had spent the last year of my life, and spent it happily too, for in every individual of his household I had seen nothing but goodness, and from them had experienced nothing but kindness and the most flattering attention.

In the doctor, extensive science, correct literary taste, and the utmost suavity and elegance of manners, are happily combined. Mrs. Cogswell has much sweetness of disposition, a highly cultivated mind, and such a dignified familiarity in her deportment as cannot fail of inspiring love and respect. When I first became acquainted with this excellent couple, they had three lovely daughters, the eldest about six years old, and the youngest, about two.

The last autumn a dreadfull disorder deprived the youngest of her hearing, and of course of the power of speech. That her life was spared, however, was an unexpected blessing, and these worthy parents received it as such. Mrs. Cogswell has lately borne the doctor a son, and their joy at this event has almost made them forget all past sorrows. It is to be regretted that this excellent mother does not enjoy, and has never enjoyed, tolerable health, as young children especially need the care of both parents. I breakfasted at the doctor's, after which I divided the forenoon between my two best friends, Henry Fish,[2] and Thomas Bull, Junr,[3] both collegiate class-mates. My Father was invited to dine at Doctor Cogswell's, and I, of course, was there too. In the afternoon, I attended the opening of the Federal-Court; took a long walk with Mr. Loomis,[4] a collegiate acquaintance, and my friend Fish; visited several of the doctor's patients; returned to my old quarters and supped; after which I spent an hour with my Father at his lodgings, where were Messrs Lynde, Clarke, and Pierpont Edwards.[5] Our conversation was desultory. Sometimes literature, and sometimes characters were the topic. Judge Edwards spoke easily and freely; but his opinions and sentiments were, manifestly, swayed by prejudice and advanced dogmatically. What a usefull and agreeable man might he be, did not his passions run away with him. About half after nine I returned to my old home, sat up an hour or two with the doctor whilst he made his charges, smoked his pipe, and read the news. I then retired to my couch and slept soundly till rather a late hour next morning.

Sabbath 18th.

After dressing, attending family duties, breakfasting etc., I waited on my Father and the other SayBrook gentlemen at their lodgings, with an offer of my services to attend them to church.

My Father accepted; but Messrs Lynde and Clarke were previously engaged to accompany Mr. Norton, their landlord. My Father and I returned to Doctor Cogswell's; sat till the bell rang; and then I waited on him and the little Misses Cogswell to their pew in the Brick-Church. We found Mr. Williams, a young divine recently settled in Mansfield, with Doctor Strong[6] in the desk. He pronounced to us one of the most finished and elegant discourses I have ever heard. His subject was the incomprehensibility of God—his Text, "Who, by searching, can find out God,"[7] or something like this. I relished the sermon much better from some small disappointment; for Judge Edwards had told me, the last evening, that none of the Williams family possessed more than ordinary talents. I did not, to be sure, altogether believe this, but I had imagined that it was not entirely without truth. I now cannot think that any of these Williamses are fools, and least of all this young preacher. The music of the day was noble and well calculated to elevate the feelings in devotion to the Almighty. This church has, probably, the best choir of singers in Connecticut; and withall a very able instructor who is constantly with them, and indeed has a salary for his support that no business may take his attention from music. Doctor Strong preached in the afternoon; and the Psalmody was even finer than in the morning.

At the third service, Parson Flint[8] made the prayers and read the Psalms, and Mr. Williams again preached. This discourse was less learned than his morning's, but not less elegantly penned, nor

6

delivered with less propriety. Elderly people in general liked it, I believe, better than the morning's. The church that we met in is a new building and a very splendid one.[9] Nothing finical about it, but it is at once beautifull and well contrived, planned, as I am told, by Mr. Daniel Wadsworth,[10] a man of strictly correct taste in architecture. Although the building is very spacious, a small, soft voice completely fills it; and the sound is not broke, as I have been led to think would, invariably, be the case, where an arch is supported by pillars with capitals. I think were Parson Hotchkiss[11] to speak in this house, all the windows would be broken; and Mr. Whittlesey's music would, undoubtedly, raise the roof.

I drank tea at Mr. Fish's and at their friendly and urgent request concluded to tarry a day or two with them. The evening passed in pleasant chat, and at a proper hour I withdrew and slept well.

Monday 19th.

I had intended, last evening, to rise early this morning, for the purpose of walking; but as I had slept little the two preceding nights, I felt too drowsy. When I went down from my chamber, I found the breakfast table set out, and the family prepared to eat. I washed, and drew up with them. Agreeable discourse with Mr. Fish gave zest to my coffee. After breakfast Henry and I employed ourselves in reading till we were pleasantly interrupted by the entrance of my Father. He did not sit long with us, however; and although the morning was excessively hot, yet my friend and I concluded to take a little exercise.

In the course of our walk I executed several little commissions; called to make enquiries after Mrs. Cogswell and her household, and was kindly reminded that my seat had been vacant at their table and was pressed to occupy it as often as I could make it agreeable. How friendly and polite is every individual of this amiable family! I have, indeed, lived with many worthy people, but never with any where every-thing was so uniformly sweetened with love and harmony.

With Henry Fish, I spent a few moments at the South-Church,

where the Freemen were holding their semi-annual meeting; but, as I hate bustles of all kinds, and especially political ones, I had not patience to stay longer. In the course of one of my last rambles for this day I called at Doctor Butler's with Homer's Iliad for Frances, a book that I had promised her the perusal of some time ago. This lady is one of four half-sisters of Mrs. Cogswell's, and a fine girl too. I wish I could be sure of as good a wife as I am confident she will make when I am disposed to marry. Drank tea with my Father at Mr. Fish's. We were all social. This family just such a one as I can be perfectly at home in. In the evening, Henry and I made a call upon Mr. Daniel Corning, who had just taken charge of the city Prison.[12] This man is an uncle of Henry's and resembles his sister, Mrs. Fish, very much, if I can judge from a miniature of her, which is said to be an excellent likeness. Mr. Corning has a frank, open countenance; and unless his face and general deportment belie him, he has a good and tender heart. I rather suspected that he had too much feeling and humanity for his station; but, on the whole, changed my opinion after having seen the firmness of his behaviour to the prisoners. I visited every apartment with him, and found some person in almost all. Among the debtors there were two or three individuals for whom every-body, almost, would have felt interested; but the appearance, and conduct, of the criminals would only have served to excite pity.

For one youth, in particular, who was imprisoned for attempting to poison an affectionate father, nothing but abhorrence could be felt. He was an only child; and the only possible motive of which I could conceive for such unnatural conduct was the hope of complete freedom from restraint; for it seems he had always been a very graceless and profligate fellow, ever impatient of the least controll or the most mild reproof. At least this was the case, as far as I could learn. He had once made considerable difficulty with the Gaoler's assistant, for which the Sherif ordered him into irons; and he was still fretfull and angry, rather than penitent, for his crime. Mr. Corning treated all very kindly; but at the same time, had so much energy, and determination in his manner as to ensure to himself full command over the most boisterous. It was easy to be seen, too, that he possessed a considerable share of *Vis-Corporis,* as well as *Vis-Mentis.* We returned to Mr. Fish's about nine; and after chatting an hour, I retired for the night.

Tuesday 20th.

A cloudy morning; my breakfast, however, relished quite as well as usual; and why should it not, for those, whose guest I was, treated me with their accustomed frankness and cordiality. About nine Henry and I walked to Doctor Cogswell's, where we spent an hour in posting his books, probably for the last time. Henry soon left me to attend some little business of his own; so, as it was rainy, I determined to seize this as an opportunity for preparing my baggage for Hanover. This occupied me till noon. Between twelve and one I sat with Mrs. Cogswell, Mrs. Daniel Wadsworth, a most charming woman, daughter to Jonathan Trumbull, and a Miss Seaber of Middletown, in whose countenance, gentleness and meekness were very strongly depicted. I think I could very well have answered for the goodness of her disposition. Between one and two, I sat down to dinner. We were all so much engaged in chat that we ate heartily almost without being aware of it. Between two and three I was present at a trifling operation performed by Doctor Cogswell in his office. The remainder of the afternoon was so unpleasant that I did not again go out, except just in the neighbourhood on an errand. I employed myself in writing, reading, and conversation with my fellow-student Nathan Strong. This gentleman was brother to my deceased friend, John McCurdy Strong, and is now the only surviving son of the old Doctor.[13] He was graduated at an early age both at Williams-College and Yale; and after spending two or three years in the study of theology, he was licensed to preach, which he did with no inconsiderable credit. On account of his youth he declined several advantageous offers of settlement; and till the year 1807 he principally spent his time in traveling through the United States, at the same time pursuing his studies; so that, at present, there is hardly a large town in the country but that he is personally acquainted in; hardly an eminent man but that he knows;

and hardly a celebrated English work but that he has perused. In addition to this, he has always had the benefit of the precepts and instructions of a father, one of the most able, independent, learned, and, I think, cunning men in Connecticut. With all these advantages, it would indeed be surprising if Mr. Strong were not a man of science and a gentleman; but notwithstanding such qualifications, I have never been pleased with him; and I believe it is generally thought that he can by no means bear comparison with his brother, a youth who was cut off in the bloom of nineteen, but who bade fair to make an eminently good as well as usefull man.

The fact is, Nature had done but little for Mr. Strong, but education, much. He will always command respect, and, as he undoubtedly has hitherto, he will continue still to deserve it.

A complaint of the lungs obliged him to give up the profession of his choice, and in the autumn of 1807 he commenced the study of medicine under Doctor Cogswell, as being in his view the next most eligible mode of life.

When Mrs. Cogswell, the young ladies, and myself sat down to tea the doctor was absent, but he soon came in.

We talked of the merits of Mr. Williams as a preacher, and as a man, and agreed that he was learned, sensible, and to all appearance good.

The doctor informed me that he spent the Sabbath-evening with him. I regretted that I did not happen to make one in the company. After tea, I amused myself with the interesting prattle of the children. How much it must add to one's happiness to be well settled in life with an amiable companion and two or three such fine children.

Wednesday 21st.

Quite an unpleasant morning—the coldest that I had remarked this season. Just after our accustomed social breakfast, Friend Fish called upon me. As this was the last day that we intended to spend in Hartford for the present, it was necessary to make many little trifling arrangements for our departure. To accomplish these, we paraded up and down Main Street at least forty times, and bustled about more than the most wealthy merchant in the place would need to in transacting the whole of his business. An errand at Daniel Hopkins' the Apothecary's; another to the Post-Office; one at Mr. Fish's store; another at Daniel Corning's shop; and last of all, a long walk with my Father up towards the north Burying-Ground pretty much finished the morning. A call upon Friend Thomas Bull and Mr. John Francis completed the forenoon and absolutely made it dinner time. Mr. Francis is the son of a respectable mechanic of Hartford, and an undergraduate at Dartmouth College. When I first entered Doctor Cogswell's office, he was at home on a visit and upon some occasion I was introduced to him. As I was now going to Hanover, it was a desirable thing to keep up his acquaintance. He gave us letters to several of his friends and acquaintances in the College; and very politely offered to render us every service in his power. Mr. Mason too, a recent graduate who was visiting Mr. Francis, did the same and also gave us letters. This gentleman belonged in west Hartford, and was now going to study theology under my cousin, Parson Witter of Wilbraham. The afternoon passed in eating peaches, apples, and pears, and in chat with Henry at his Father's. In the beginning of the evening we waited on Doctors Cogswell and Sparhawk[14] for our introductory letters and received one from each of the gentlemen addressed to Doctor Nathan Smith. Doctor Sparhawk was educated under Professor Smith and had recently settled in Hartford. About eight o'clock I accompanied Henry to return a book to Mr. Daniel Danforth's, a merchant in Burr Street. I should have been happy to spend the evening there but Miss Montague, Mrs. Danforth's sister, whose company would have been the principal inducement, was out. Of this young lady, I know but little, except that she has the most interesting face I have ever seen. The expression of it is precisely like that of John McCurdy Strong's; and this expression is the only thing in which the portrait that I have of that valued friend is deficient.

I first saw Miss Montague during an illness through which Doctor Cogswell attended her as physician. At this time, I thought her a handsome girl, but a few months afterwards, meeting her at the bed-side of a brother who was dangerously sick, I was struck with her resemblance to Strong. Since that time I have met her often; and I can confidently say that no lady of my acquaintance possesses a face and person any where near so pleasing and agreeable to me as hers. I hope her mind is as well cultivated, and her heart as good as Frances Butler's (and I am sure, from her manners, they may very well be so), and then I should hardly know which to recommend, most highly, to my best friend, in case he should want a wife. Give *her*, who is destined to be my companion for life, Miss Montague's person and face and Miss Butler's mind and qualifications, and I shall, most willingly, resign to others all the Belles of the present Age.[15]

Thursday 22nd.

This morning rose uncommonly early, though the stage did not leave town till eight, and I had made every necessary preparation for my journey the preceding day. When I am going any where, especially if I am to start early in the day, I have long remarked that I am less drowsy in the morning than usual; and so it happened in this case. Whether the anticipated pleasure refreshes the system and makes sleep less necessary; or whether it enables us to sleep at a greater rate than ordinary, I shall not pretend to determine; but the fact is certain that I was, this morning, awake long enough before the day began to dawn; and notwithstanding my better judgment pointed out the folly of it I could not forbear to paint Hanover, and Dartmouth-College, in the colours of New Haven, and Yale. I was utterly unable to persuade myself but that the scenes of my past collegiate life would again be renewed, and my heart warmed at the bare recollection of my winter evenings at Yale where every social affection was brought into action by the companions of my choice, and the friends of my highest regard. The memory of Strong rushed forcibly upon me; and my heart felt a pang for his loss. Peace to his ashes! His virtues would have graced a cottage, or expanded the breast of a prince. His amiableness of deportment and sweetness of disposition would have ensured him the love of all his acquaintance.

At Yale I first had the happiness of knowing him. There, he became my friend, and there, "First my heart to sacred Friendship beat." He was just maturing to usefullness. Elegant in his person and manners; with a mind liberal and well-cultivated, he was snatched from all who held him dear on earth. The attachment of his numerous friends was ardent, and would have been lasting. The affection of his brother and sister for him was, no doubt, unbounded. His only surviving parent doated on him. On him he placed all his reliance for consolation and support in his old age. Many were the hearts that were wrung at his melancholy death. How often have I contemplated his blooming similitude, and almost forgot that it is all I shall ever more behold of him. Vain, indeed, was the hope of finding, in such a place as Dartmouth, and in one short year, a companion like him.

My Father was invited to breakfast with us; and he made his appearance soon after the family were up. Our conversation, of course, turned upon the place whither we were going, and the time of our absense. Six months, I thought, was as little as it would be worth while to go so great a distance for; especially as I conceived that a person could not but study advantageously under the instructor of such a Medical School. I was aware that I could have the benefit of but little practice; but the advantage that must result from seeing dissections, and from having access to a complete Anatomical-Museum, would be much greater than what I could expect from any instructor in Connecticut. Besides, from the best information I could obtain, the expence of living at Hanover was likely to be as little, and even less, than in eligible places in my native state. Thus, economy and improvement presented a double inducement to spend the winter under Dr. Smith.

Whilst we were at table, Mr. Francis entered with two or three letters more, and just as we rose, Thomas Bull made a call. Neither of these gentlemen staid long. I made arrangements, however, with Thomas, for the transmission of our letters; for though we had talked upon this before, yet we had not absolutely determined upon any way. Thomas had been in his father's store till now, ever since he took his degree; but on coming to age was just going to set up for himself at so great a distance from home as

New-Connecticut.[16] After parting with him I went to take leave of Dr. Cogswell's family. From having lived so long and so harmoniously with them, and from knowing the peculiar delicacy of their feelings upon such occasions, I considered this as quite a task; and accordingly, resolved to get through it as quickly as possible. The servants I bade a good morning with as pleasant a face as I could assume; I kissed the children; shook hands with Mrs. Cogswell and the doctor; bade them all adieu, and turned abruptly off. The doctor and Mrs. Cogswell possess exquisite sensibility. The tears started in their eyes. I, on my part, could not but feel a great deal of regret at parting with persons whom I revered and loved as I do every individual of this excellent family; but my feelings, I suppose, are much less acute on such occasions than most people's. I went, immediately, to the stage-house and found all waiting for the mail. My Father staid till the stage drew up. It was nine o'clock before I shook hands with him and got well seated in it. There were five or six passengers, but only one who seemed inclined to contribute to any-body's amusement. His name was Brewster, and he seemed to be a man who had acquired considerable information by extensive intercourse through the country; and by having seen much of what is called good company. He made considerable pretensions to correct taste in some branches of literature; but it was easy to see that the sphere of his book knowledge was very contracted and that he was best calculated to shine as a horse-jockey. I, as usual, when riding felt but little inclined to be talkative; but Mr. Brewster named Doctor Dwight,[17] and about him I was willing to converse. He was mentioned, in very exalted terms, as a scholar and an agreeable man, but Mr. Brewster thought him enthusiastic. Many anecdotes illustrative of his character were related, and on the whole time passed agreeably.

Our route lay through Windsor, the oldest town in the State; but not so interesting to me from that circumstance as from its being a very handsome place and the residence of my Friend Elisha Beebe Strong,[18] a gentleman who belonged to the freshman-class in Yale College during the last year that I spent there, and who was introduced to my acquaintance by Mr. Fish. His exteriour was elegant, his manners engaging, and his disposition open and friendly; and a considerable intimacy took place between us. I have seen him seldom since I left New-Haven, but, when we have met, he has always appeared to be the same pleasant & frank-hearted fellow that he formerly was.

His Father's seat in Windsor is handsome, but not splendid. I had only a passing view of it, but I did not see a more pleasant situation in the town.

Dr. Wolcott's[19] next attracted my attention; but there was nothing remarkable pertaining to it except the good man its master. The appearance of the house and grounds that once belonged to Judge Elsworth,[20] I had often admired; and they appeared now no less pleasant than formerly.

We reached Suffield at eleven. This town adjoins Windsor. Here we were to dine, and, on account of the Distributing-Post-Office, to be detained till two or three o'clock. The stage-house was kept by Joseph Utley, formerly of Hartford, in whose family I recollected that Aunt Ely had once been intimate. I saw nobody except himself, one daughter, and a servant or two. Soon after we alighted, a coach drove up that left Hartford about the time that we did. It belonged to General Stephen Row Bradley,[21] L.L.D. Dartmuthensis, of Vermont, and contained him, his wife, his son's wife, and their attendants. The General came directly into the bar-room, where he soon showed himself to be a right tavern-politician. If this man sustains the whole dignity of Vermont in our legislature, I think it cannot be very burthensome. Just as General Bradley rode off, who should come up but Justin Lyman[22] of New-York, a man born in Vermont, but a resident of Hartford till quite lately. He was bred a merchant, but is now, exactly, one of Salmagundi's little great men. He is never so happy as when surrounded by a cluster of the most ragged of the *Sovereign People,* who shall be disposed to stand, with open mouths, listening to his harangues. I think if he were obnoxious to any Government, the best way of getting rid of him would be to give him an office, which, I am sure, would puff him up so much that he would ultimately burst. Mr. Lyman staid to dinner, & at table took upon himself to be the oracle of the company. Mr. Atwater,[23] of New-Haven, soon drove up and joined us. He was accompanied by his wife and another lady. This old gentleman was formerly Steward to Yale-College; and, as every-body else would have done in his station, he gave great *dis*satisfaction.

I remember having heard that the students, upon some occasion whilst the Commons were under his direction, had half-baked bread set before them upon which two or three tables joined and made a small image out of it to represent the Devil; out of whose mouth hung a paper, inscribed with these words: "Give an account of thy Stewardship; for thou canst, no longer, be Steward." This was placed, over night, upon the steps of the old gentleman's door, so as to present itself the first thing in the morning.

I was told that this little trick operated, quite powerfully, upon his feelings. Mr. Atwater had now, probably, been visiting his friends in Massachusetts and was returning home.

Our dinner was good. I could find fault in but one particular; and that was we were obliged to sit in too crowded a manner at the table. After we rose, we had abundant leisure to view Mr. Granger's[24] seat, which was directly across the street from us, and to speculate upon peddling feathers and wooden-bowls; topics that the place in which we were naturally suggested.

In the afternoon, Utley's daughter took a seat with us in the stage for the first town in Massachusetts. As we were all strangers to her, she spoke little. About half a mile above Suffield-Post-Office we took in a young couple, whom I should have judged, from behavior, to be brother and sister had they in the least resembled each other. Both appeared to be under twenty. The female was entirely silent the whole afternoon; but the gentleman, quite talkative. His name, we soon learned, was Lovel, and a native of Rockingham in Vermont, whither he was now returning from an excursion into Connecticut. Mr. Lovel seemed to be an honest, good-hearted fellow; but necessarily, from what I supposed had been his education, somewhat simple. His countenance was good and on the whole interesting, for, though I could not help smiling many times at him, yet I felt quite prepossessed in his favour; and at parting I wanted, very much, to have further opportunity of knowing him. We reached Pomeroy's Tavern,[25] in North-Hampton, about seven P.M. and were informed that we should start early next morning. I regretted this, as I was quite curious to see the place that had given to our *Alma Mater, Yalensia,* her President; a man of whom all Connecticut justly feels *Proud*; a man who has fortitude and integrity enough to break with his dearest bosom friends,[26] when they adopt principles subversive of the religion of his blessed Master, and of course, subversive of all good order and moral obligation; to break with these friends although they are men of great worldly power, and in high honour among men. Mr. Brewster left us at this house. Our party at supper consisted of Mr. Lovel, and his companion, another gentleman, that had accompanied us from Hartford but had not spoken during the whole ride except to give a negative or affirmative (and that in a very low voice) to questions that were put to him by Mr. Fish, and myself. We were convinced before we rose from the table that our silent companion was either *non compos mentis* or a hypochondriac.

The Supreme Court of Massachusetts happened at this time to be in session, and, in consequence of it, the house where we were was much crowded with company that were brought together on the occasion. I should have passed the evening very unpleasantly, had not a gentleman, soon after supper, entered whom I directly understood to be Ebenezer Hunt,[27] M.D., a man whose conversation would amuse and instruct for any length of time. I listened to him with peculiar pleasure; for, from his being a particular friend of Doctor Cogswell, I had often heard the excellence of his character. He is a man of about fifty; six feet in height; athletic, and well-formed in every limb, and with a mind, strong, well cultivated; and all in proportion to his appearance. He has long been the principal man in the large County of Hampshire and has undeniably merited every honour that has been confered upon him. A few moments after he retired, a class mate, whom I had not seen since we parted at Yale, entered and greeted me most cordially. It was Edmund Bliss,[28] of Springfield, the most eccentric character of my acquaintance. Whenever he chose, he could make any person who knew him ever so well believe that black was white; and with these talents, so well adapted to the profession he was studying: the Law. His business at Northampton at this time was, of course, to attend the court. Mr. Bliss tarried about half an hour and then withdrew. When arrangements were to be made for accommodating us with beds, it appeared that our female-fellow-passenger was Mrs. Lovel. What awkwardnesses does traveling in the stage occasion a new-married couple. I think I shall always contrive, in similar circumstances, to travel in a private chaise or stay at home.

On account of the crowd in the house previous to our coming, our accommodations were not quite so pleasant as they would, perhaps, otherwise have been; but, on the whole, we did tolerably well. Friend Fish and I were now bed-fellows for the first time since we lived together at New-Haven.

Fryday 23rd.

Arose early, and waited long and impatiently for breakfast. Did not get away so soon, by an hour and a half, as I expected; but when we did start, our ride was pleasant and was through several fine and beautiful villages. We dined at Greenfield, a place for which I could not but feel a kind of regard on account of its namesake, in Connecticut, which has been the subject of a very charming poem.[29] We staid a long time at this place; but, on the whole, spent it agreeably, for we found a back-gammon-table at the house where we were, and with that Henry and I diverted ourselves. I should, to be sure, have prefered walking about and viewing the town, but we were in momentary expectation of being summoned to our seats in the stage, and we did not, on that account, like to be out of the way. Our company here was the same that it had been all the way from Hartford, with the exception of Mr. Brewster, who, I have before mentioned, left us at North-Hampton. The silent man concluded to tarry here.

The stage-drivers in Massachusetts, I remark, are in much less haste to accomplish their day's journey than those I have ridden with in Connecticut, and much more complaisant to persons whom they meet. There is more need of all this, however, as the roads are not so good.

We got into Vermont early in the afternoon, for we had not yet crossed the river. At Guilford we took into the stage for a few miles a tailoress, as I judged by her press-board and goose. She was certainly Mrs. Grumley's daughter, if there is any judging by resemblance. As soon as I entered Vermont, I saw children by dozens, lads with squirrels tails for feathers; and girls with snake-skins for sashes. The country, very rough. Dropped directly down into Brattleborough, where we were to tarry for the night. Remembered that I had scarcely seen the Connecticut since we left Hartford, and yet supposed we must have traveled all the way at no great distance from it. The road, after we entered Vermont, was very dreary. No steeples, or churches, to be seen.

One thing, however, that served to make the ride tolerable was the purchase of about a peck of pears of an old lady that lived by the road side. We had the consolation, too, in this state not to be stopped very frequently by post-offices. We found General Bradley again in this place; and I believe he tarried all night, though, as we had a room pretty much to ourselves did not see him in the course of the evening. Heard his character of a New-Hantonian,[30] who accidentally put up with us, and found he was just such a man as I had judged him to be. The stranger and I had much conversation. We spoke of the several states in the union, and, among the rest, of my native one. He considered it as the most learned and refined, and, of course, the most liberal and happy, in the country. As I had formerly been so little out of Connecticut, I had never before heard any thing said of it; and this was only the opinion of an individual, but as he did not know where I belonged I considered it as his true opinion, and I was accordingly much gratified with it. Whilst we were at supper, a gentleman arrived in the northern stage and joined us. He was mighty solicitous for news from Boston—mighty pompous and important too. No great things like small potatoes, thought I. Montes parturiunt. When he left the room, I was informed that he was a Boston-bankrupt.

Henry and I retired together, quite early, and slept tolerably.

Saturday 24th.

Was called up in the morning at the hour of three, but the stage did not get away till the hour of four. The carriage in which we rode was narrow and short, and this morning, as well as the last, was cold and blustering. A heavy fog, in addition to all this, incommoded us much.

From Westminster we crossed the Connecticut, for the first time, and found ourselves in Walpole, New-Hampshire. In quite a central part of this town we stopped to take breakfast.

I remarked, directly across the way from the stage-house, the Office of the Political Observatory,[31] which was once managed by Stanley Griswold, the renegade clergyman from Connecticut, who was afterwards appointed to some public office in the North-western-territory by the President, but has, recently, been turned from it for breach of trust. I think I could be willing for the sake of the good people of Connecticut that New-Hampshire should have Whitfield Cowles to look out from this self-same observatory.

Walpole, quite an elegant little village. After breakfast stepped across the way to a merchant's, Mr. Sparhawk, for whom I had letters. They were from his brother, Dr. Sparhawk, of Hartford, and were put into my hands not long before I left that place. At Walpole, Mr. Lovel and his wife left us, after expressing wishes to Mr. Fish and me for further acquaintance and inviting us to visit them, if we should ever come to Rockingham. Their places were filled by a young student of Dartmouth, a member of the junior-class. His name was Charles Adams,[32] and he appeared to be a very sprightly, intelligent fellow. We dined at Windsor. This [is] another handsome place, and withall the residence of Bancroft Fowler,[33] now a clergyman, but formerly a Tutor in Yale. At Charlestown, between Walpole and Windsor, we took in several students; and at Windsor again, another, a Mr. Curtiss, brother-in-law to Parson Fowler. With Curtiss I was much pleased, but the rest had nothing remarkable about them.

When we came out from dinner, we found already seated in the stage a stranger with a wife and child or two, and a Captain Grant. These accompanied us to Hanover, and made our number in the whole twelve. Saw Mr. Park somewhere in Windsor Street, but did not have opportunity to speak with him. This gentleman I became acquainted with whilst living in Doctor Bacon's family. He was born of indigent parents in Connecticut but had removed, some time since, into Michilimakinak, where he attracted the notice of some gentleman who was so convinced of his talents and genius that he determined to give him an education at Dartmouth. He was a senior at the time of his visiting Hartford; in which place the letters that he brought insured him a welcome reception. Our driver this afternoon did not hasten, and the shades of night overspread us before we had gone over two thirds the remaining distance. The whole route was Terra Incognita to me. The road was sometimes level, and sometimes hilly; sometimes rough, and sometimes smooth. We were, occasionally, on the east side of the Connecticut, and, occasionally, on the west. Sometimes, I imagined we were going South, and sometimes, North. To be sure, our conversation in some measure beguiled us of the tediousness of the way, for from the circumstance that Captain Grant was a native of Connecticut we talked of that place; and the students, occasionally, put in questions about our College, its situation, its officers, studies, and laws. The manners and customs of the people of our large towns, and those of our farmers, were described and compared; and all the New-England states were, in their turns, our topics. About nine we arrived at Dewey's Tavern,[34] in Hanover, and very joyfully allighted in hopes of pleasant accommodations. On entering the house, a sour landlord, and a very dirty bar room full of persons of all descriptions met our sight. I soon perceived that our quarters were not likely to be very agreeable; but I hoped not to be driven to the necessity of changing them, either at a late hour on Saturday night or on the Sabbath. I was disappointed, however, in this expectation; for, although we made shift to put up with much incivility before and during supper, yet when we requested beds, we received such treatment that we resolved to take our baggage and seek a more hospitable roof. Captain Grant had not staid, even to sit, in the house; but the students, who were our fellow travellers, supped with us. One who was a candidate for the sophomore class and who belonged to Salem, from not having been in the place before was unprovided with quarters in the College, or else where, and accompanied us to another tavern; but the rest dispersed different ways to their acquaintance. A man that was passing, just as we got into the street, directed us to Bush's Hotel. Mr. Bush[35] was a graduate of the College, and from that circumstance I expected gentlemanly treatment, though we had failed of receiving it from a Deacon of the Church. He met us at the door with a pleasant countenance, and we entered a spacious, ill contrived, unfinished, and uncleanly house. It did not appear to be nigh so well ordered as most farmer's houses in Connecticut; but we were, at this time, in a humour to put up with almost any-thing. We applied for beds. All he had were occupied, except two in one chamber. Mr. Fish and I would have prefered a room to ourselves on account of conversation; but as we liked our companion very-well, and especially, as it would have been to no purpose to make objections to this arrangement, we cheerfully accepted the offered accommodations, such as they were. Our beds were tolerably clean and comfortable, considering where we obtained them; and, after a short conversation on Deacon Dewey's inhospitality, we fell asleep.

Sabbath 25th.

This morning I awoke, long before my Friend Fish and even before daylight. I reflected, with considerable dissatisfaction, on my reception, and subsequent entertainment, in Hanover.

I had, to be sure, come to the place not for the purpose of polishing my manners, but with a view of improving my mind by a course of Dr. Smith's Lectures. I had no personal knowledge of my intended instructor, nor till now of the town; but I had understood from Messrs Hunt[36] and Simmons[37] that they were well satisfied with both. The correctness of their judgment respecting one I now began to doubt; and as they could not be very well qualified from their educations to judge of the other I almost suspected their opinions were, on both points, erroneous.

I had, indeed, been in but two houses; but it was fair to form judgment of the rest from these, as they were the two best public-houses in Town. One of the landlords, too, had been liberally educated; and of course his advantages for becoming polite had been greater than I could suppose the advantages of others had been. How is it possible, thought I, that there should not be wealth and refinement where so many gentlemen from large towns are, constantly, going and coming. If the people are not absolutely stupid, surely they would have caught at least one particle of liberality. When I got up, I found the house quite as slovenly as it appeared last night. The weather was rainy, and I found no pleasant corner within doors, and no tolerable walking, without. Breakfast was not prepared till a late hour; and when we were ushered to the table, we found it coarsely set, and without a cloth. Captain Grant, who had left Dewey's before supper last evening; Mr. Prescott,[38] a medical student of no very prepossessing exteriour, but really an agreeable clever fellow, and Mr. Trask[39] another young physician and quite a gentleman in manners and dress, together with the sophomore candidate, Mr. Fish, and myself made up our whole party. Every thing upon the table was answerable to the general appearance of the house, not even excepting our landlady, whom I do not hesitate to pronounce a slut. No wonder our appetites were not good. When we rose, Mr. Fish and I, notwithstanding the rain, took our umbrellas and walked across the public-area. The College, on the east-side, attracted our attention first. It is a neat and really handsome building, and as well situated as it can be in Hanover. It is three stories high; perhaps a hundred and fifty feet long; forty wide; built of wood; ornamented with a cupula; and neatly painted, with white-lead. At the southwest corner of this edifice, and in front of it, stands the chapel, a square, two-story house with quite a flat roof. This very much disfigures the appearance of the College. Directly south of the chapel, stands the President's House, which is neat, not elegant. On the north side of the green stand two handsome dwelling-houses and a decent church. On the west, the most elegant house in the town. These, with two or three stores and a few other, shabby, old broken-windowed buildings, make the place. The green, I should judge to be but little short of a quarter of a mile square, and is uneven, with roads crossing it diagonally. It is uninclosed, as is the College-Yard. Roads go out of the town from the four corners of this area; and on all of them are a few moderate-looking houses. The face of the country was both uneven and rough.

The horizon was very circumscribed; and on which side so ever I turned my eyes I beheld one hill, rising above another, all covered with the trunks of large trees over which the fire had passed. What was called Hanover plain (which, by the by, I venture to say is more rough than any spot in Connecticut) was varigated with burnt shrubs, rocks and stones, virginia, and crag-fences. The unpleasantness of the weather, the aspect of the place and its vicinity, and the strange singularity of the people altogether disgusted me, and twenty-times I wished myself at home, even without knowing anything of Doctor Smith, or the College-Institution. After our ramble, we seated ourselves in Esquire Bush's best room, and for want of something better, read news-papers for pastime till the second ringing of the bell for church. We attended, of course, and were waited upon and shown to seats by Messrs Prescot and Trask. Divine service was performed by Mr. Shurt[l]iff,[40] Professor of Theology in the College, the people of the town being too indigent to settle a clergyman. The preacher's face indicated goodness, rather than greatness. There was nothing in it, however, inconsistent with a sound mind and extensive science. The man's whole appearance was mild and winning. The sermon was ordinary, but it was extemporaneous. I was willing to make allowance for this, as I was told he had, for the week past, been closely and indispensably engaged in the business of the College. The audience consisted of about twenty persons, half of which number were, probably, students. Five men made up the whole choir of singers; one of which officiated as Chorister and accompanied the rest on a bass-viol. Their tunes were Old Hundred, Mear, and one or two more, far inferiour to these. The performance was, on the whole, much better than could, under existing circumstances, have been well expected.

We dined in much the same style that we breakfasted in, and with the same company, though, as we were more hungry, the dinner relished a little better.

I began now to be some acquainted with the medical students; and of course to be social. I mentioned Doctor Smith but was informed that he was out of town. I enquired if any medical students were here from Connecticut. It was believed that there was a Yale-graduate in the place and that his name was Atwater,[41] but no one was acquainted with him or could tell where he lodged. I supposed this gentleman must be Mr. William Atwater, a native of the south of Massachusetts, nephew to the old gentleman whom we met on the road up, and the person who took a degree in the year 1807. He had never been a particular acquaintance of mine, though I had long known him and respected him for scholarship. Our present circumstances, of course, removed all distance that in any other situation might have taken place between us; and I must confess that in the afternoon I went to church, through all the rain, merely in the hope of meeting him. Service had just commenced when, casting my eyes around, he met my sight though, apparently, without noticing me. When we were dismissed from the house, however, he very cordially greeted Mr. Fish and me, expressing much joy at seeing us, as he had already been a week in the place, and had spent it quite as solitarily as we had one day. He accompanied us to our lodgings, where after having a fire made up, we sat down and had an agreeable chat about old friends, New Haven, Yale College, and so forth; and all this, notwithstanding the two medical students, the young sophomore, and Captain Grant were present. I believe they thought us very ostentatious, for in the course of our conversation we gave a complete history of the persons, characters, and functions of President Dwight and his Faculty. These topics were, naturally, the first to present themselves, as all our acquaintance, hitherto, with Mr. Atwater had been at New Haven; and we were less considerate about indulging ourselves upon them, as we had been so lonesome ever since we had left home. Mr. Atwater insisted on retiring at tea-time, but promised to call and spend the evening in our company.

Our supper was served up on the same uncovered table that we had before ate upon; but it had, in the mean time, been pretty copiously rubbed over with some very fetid oil. Our fare was Bohea tea, and brown sugar, a rye-toast, without plates or forks, and some tolerably good cheese.

We were more sociable at this meal than at any previous one, and I, for my part, was much pleased, both with Prescott and Trask. The young sophomore was certainly a clever fellow, and Grant laid himself out for ours and his own entertainment. This last mentioned gentleman, it seemed, had been bred a printer; but prefering the life of a sailor, he had followed the seas, till Mr. Jefferson's embargo threw him out of business. As his education had been a good common one, he was now engaged to conduct the Hanover-Gazette by its proprietor. Mr. Atwater was punctual to his appointment, and our evening passed in more general sociality. When conversation near the close of the evening began to droop a little, I mentioned Salmagundi,[42] which I had brought for the purpose of reading it in the stage. All had heard of the work, but none had seen it; so, as literature had been our subject hitherto, I deemed it proper that we should close our discourses with some literary production. Mr. Atwater and I read alternately, to general entertainment, as all professed. Those that I thought the most laughable pieces were chosen; and at the end of each, we severally made our remarks. We broke up our party at a late hour, and from the pleasantness of this evening, I felt somewhat reconciled to Hanover. Mr. Atwater, before he retired, pressingly invited Mr. Fish and me to make his room our own till we could settle ourselves, which we agreed to do.

So much for the longest journey that I ever took in my life, the object of which was not to visit friends. By the way, I expected no pleasure, and found much; in Hanover, I expected to see elegance, and refinement, and was disappointed. When I was disgusted with the place and the people and heartily wished myself at home, I found a friend in whose company I could, at any period and for any length of time, be entertained and happy.

May these little incidents teach me wisdom; guard me against vain expectations; and warn me against making myself unhappy at disappointment, "The Lot of Man."

N.B. This Journal is to be continued in another Volume.

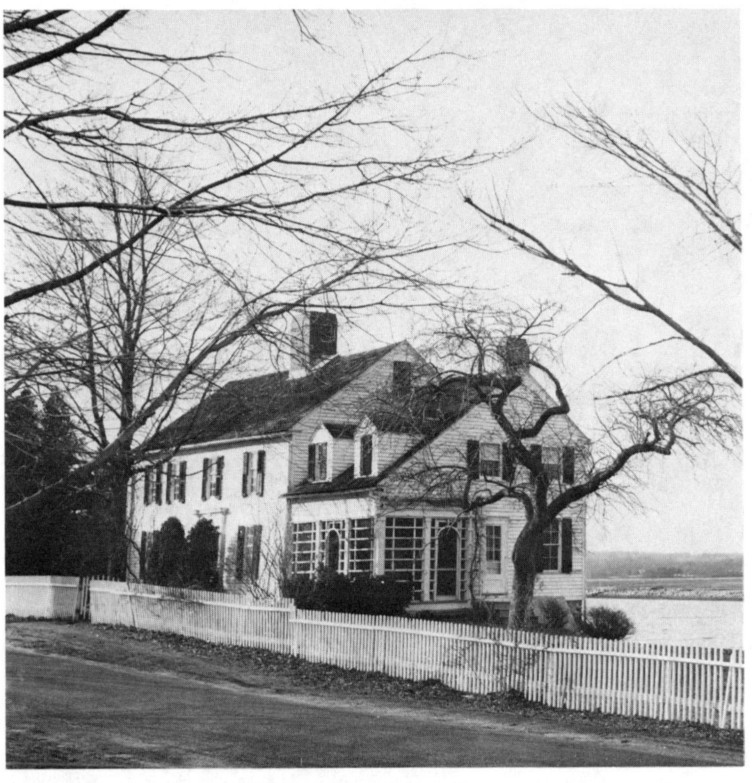

William Tully's birthplace. The house, built by his grandfather, is still standing on North Cove, Saybrook Point, Connecticut. *Photograph by Herbert Thoms, M.D.*

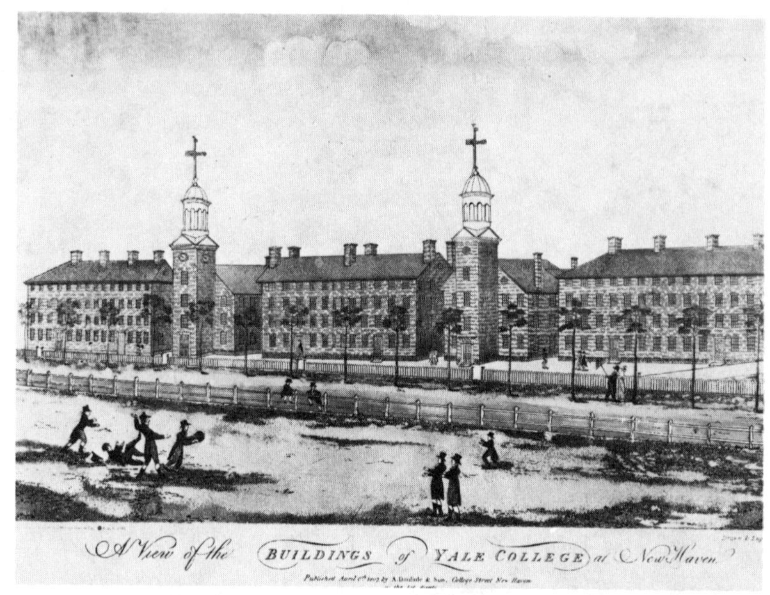

This view of Yale College in 1807 by Amos Doolittle shows the five southernmost buildings of the Old Brick Row facing the New Haven Green. *Yale University Archives, Yale University Library.*

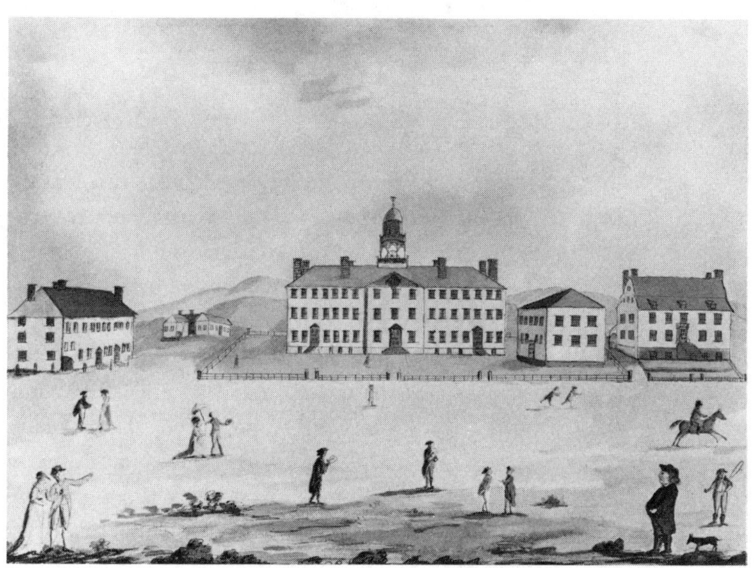

A view of the main building of Dartmouth College and the Chapel at
the right by George Tichnor in 1803. *Courtesy of the Dartmouth
College Library.*

JOURNAL

Awoke early, as usual, and found the day even more unpleasant and cold than the preceding. We had been informed on the Sabbath that Doctor N. Smith, to whom our letters were directed, was out of town and quite a disappointment it was to us; but this morning at breakfast, we learned, with much pleasure, that he had returned. Before we rose from the table, Mr. Atwater entered; and after cordial salutations, he again entreated us to make his room our home till we could get settled; and he proffered his service in assisting us to obtain lodging and boarding, and to wait on us to Doctor Smith's. The latter offer we immediately accepted, and off we marched to call on our instructor that was to be. After rapping almost all the skin from our knuckles, we were at last heard, and bade to walk in, but the Doctor was out. After loitering about the street awhile, we called again and found him. He is a man of medium height, rather thin, and spare; his dress was quite plain, very heedlessly chosen, and carelessly put on. He received us in a blunt but civil way and, on the whole, his appearance and manner was much like a Connecticut farmer. He took our letters, which were from Drs. Cogswell and Sparhawk, and after reading them, told us that he was pleased we had come just at this time as he hoped his present course of lectures would be superiour to any former one; adding that he had engaged a Dr. Ramsay,[43] of Edinburgh, to give a course on Anatomy and Physiology. Thought I, we are not likely to be burdened with compliments, for, all this while, he had not introduced us to the ladies of his family, and three were sitting, silently, engaged in some kind of needlework. There was, likewise, in the room one gentleman, whom I judged to be a medical student that boarded in his family, and two lads that were probably his sons. We discoursed awhile respecting the Lectures, till at Last the Doctor enquired about Professor Sil[l]iman.[44]

Of him, he spoke as the first chemist in New-England; and told us that after hearing a course from such a man, with such an apparatus as he possessed, he deemed himself unable, under his circumstances, to be of much service to us in that branch.

The Doctor remarked further that he meddled with chemistry only because there was nobody else to treat of the subject, and he considered it as the foundation of Medicine.

He next enquired if we had obtained a room and place to board; and on our answering in the negative, he kindly offered, in consideration of our being strangers in the place, to take on himself the burthen of doing this. We made our acknowledgments for his politeness and gratefully accepted his offer. After telling us to come and dine with him, he withdrew to attend his business; and we walked from his house to Mr. Atwater's room, where we chatted pleasantly, till Dr. Smith unexpectedly found us and gave notice that he was ready to introduce us to the best quarters he could obtain in the place. They were in a neighbouring tavern; and we were to have a furnished room, board, lodging, and washing, at two dollars fifty cents a week. We were not much pleased with our landlord's appearance; but because Doctor Smith had got us into his family, we concluded it to be a good place. Mr. Fish and I resolved to take possession the following afternoon and so returned to Mr. Atwater's room. At one, the hour of dinner, we called at Mr. Smith's. The same persons were in his house that we had seen in the morning, the two lads excepted, but yet no introduction. The table was all spread, and he at once invited us to draw up, which we accordingly did, without blessing, or even compliments, of any kind.

The food was nicely dressed and wholesome, consisting of beef, pork, and vegetables, of various kinds, all served up in farmer's way. The Doctor helped himself, and requested us to do the same. Nobody seemed disposed to introduce a conversation, and I took the liberty to mention the intended medical establishment at Yale.[45] The Doctor enquired particularly respecting it, and thought the plan, on the whole, quite a liberal one. He remarked that in this part of the country such a setting out would be deemed quite extravagant. He gave it as his opinion that medical-societies, though their intention may be good, generally fall so far short of their proposed object as to do more hurt than good; and he felt convinced that Yale would do better without assistance from any such Institution.[46] He further added that *he* had not only been destitute of patronage of that kind, but had been unable to obtain assistance from the state; and that the College had done nothing more than lend him their name.

Literary-establishments, he remarked, never flourished, unless their instructors depended upon their own exertions for support. Legislatures ought to make donations for buildings and apparatus; but the emolument to the teacher ought to come from the pupils; the number of which, of course, depends upon his reputation. Harvard-University was named as an example of the ruinous effects of funds for the support of the faculty of the Institution, as it had been making no improvements since about the year 1750.[47] The medical professors now read the same lectures, verbatim, that they did twenty or thirty years ago. Yale he considered as now having the preeminence of every college in the country, and, as in the fairest way to preserve it, especially should Dr. Dwight be spared long enough to put his many excellent plans for its improvement into execution. After dinner I returned to Mr. Atwater's room and of him learned the following particulars. Dr. Smith, in early life, had nothing more than a common education till, at the age of 18, or 19, he put himself under a country physician and qualified himself, as others of his time did, for the practice of medicine.

After this, he settled in Windsor, Vermont[48]; but found himself, as he imagined, so deficient that he determined, as soon as he could raise money enough, to study a year or two at Harvard. He accordingly did but, in proportion as he acquired information, his desire for it increased, and from Harvard he removed to Columbia-College,[49] in New-York, and thence to the celebrated University in Edinburgh. On his return to his native country, he found himself several thousand dollars in debt, but with unwearied industry he has since laboured till he has cancelled every pecuniary obligation; though his creditors, as long as he had any, constantly embarrassed him. He now posesses quite a handsome little estate. At Dartmouth-College he set himself up; purchased his own apparatus; and till within a year, he has never had any other assistance than just the countenance of the College. His students are now, annually, about fifty; and his school is really at present the second[50] in the country.

On calling, this afternoon, upon Mr. Chandler,[51] our landlord that was to be, we found that since his agreement with Dr. Smith he had determined to afford us nothing but an unfurnished room and board for the price talked of. We thought him both fraudulent and exhorbitant; and, as we had never liked either him or the appearance of the inside of his house, we very easily resolved to have nothing more to do with him. We could not now think of again giving Dr. Smith the trouble of negotiating for us; so we set off ourselves in quest of quarters.

After application at every possible place, we were unsuccessfull, for either every room was engaged, or occupied, or those that intended to rent chambers were keeping them till the demand should be greater in hopes of an unreasonable price.

From the littleness and narrowness of disposition that was so manifest in every person to whom we applied, we did not hesitate to decide that the latter was the cause of our disappointment. We now concluded that we should most certainly be under the necessity of returning to Connecticut, merely because this paltry little village, in which the College never ought to have been placed, would not entertain us reasonably for a few months. It was evident that if the inhabitants had ever possessed one single spark of manhood, or enterprise, they might, honourably, have become rich from the wealth that the students, and the collegiate festivals, had brought into the place. From information, however, that we had received from our friends, we might have expected to find in the Hanoverians, a people calculating to live as parsimoniously as possible, without any regard to the comforts of life—to entertain a stranger as miserably as he will put up with, and for the greatest possible price that can be extorted from him—too lazy to make any exertions of their own but depending entirely upon the College for support; and withall too ignorant to have any idea of a better possible mode of life. This we had looked upon as a carricature, delineated by the pencil of prejudice and enmity; but now, as far as our knowledge extended (and it was to all the common people of the place), we found the likeness true and accurate in every particular. Notwithstanding all our dissatisfaction and mortification, since we reached Hanover, we had received evidence of the excellence of Doctor Smith; and we had not the least reason to suppose but that his lectures would be quite as good as common fame represented them. In addition to this, we had come two hundred miles, and should we, by immediately returning home, make so long a journey but a fool's errand? This question, which we had more than once put to ourselves, now recurred so forcibly that we resolved to try, once more, to come to terms with Mr. Chandler. All our endeavors, however, were in vain, for the man was even more unreasonable than before; and we left him, disgusted with his meanness and illiberality. Our evening passed, in a tolerably pleasant manner, at Bush's in company with Captain Grant, a Mr. Smith, and two men, who, we found, had once belonged to East-Haddam in Connecticut. Of Mr. Smith, we knew nothing; but, from his conversation we judged that he had once been a member of the College but was now a merchant in Boston. Business had brought him to Hanover, and as the stage did not leave the place but once in a week, he was compelled to tarry here several days. Grant and he seemed to be old acquaintances, so were, of course, talkative enough. The other two men, I conjectured, were farmers who had removed into Vermont, but what brought them to Hanover, I believe was known only to themselves.

We retired at a late hour, and slept as well as could be expected in Hanover.

Tuesday 27th.

Awoke early; but as I had no particular employment, and the beds were the best things I had seen in the place, I determined, if it may be so termed, to indulge myself till a late hour. In another

34

bed that stood in our chamber, which the two last nights had been occupied by the young sophomore heretofore mentioned, now slept a medical-student, by the name of Sartwell,[52] & an undergraduate named Sprague. Sartwell, on horseback, had rode, in company with the stage, a considerable distance whilst we were in Massachusetts; but, it seemed, had just now reached Hanover. Sprague had taken seat with us at Charlestown; and I then decided him to be, in disposition, though not in talents, another *Ben. Carnes.*[53] How he came to be here this night, I am unable to say. Last evening he had requested to be waked to prayers, in case the bell should be heard; and now, as I desired to talk with Henry, I determined that it should not be my fault if we did not get rid of him at the time he seemed solicitous to go. Accordingly, I took care that he should leave us soon; as did Sartwell, after some general conversation on collegiate affairs, and the difficulty of obtaining accommodations in Hanover.

Mr. Fish and I then agreed that from what we had seen of Chandler, we would not at any rate live in his house, but thought it best to make reasonable exertion during the day for a room, and if unsuccessfull, to take the next stage for Connecticut. With these resolutions, we rose, found the same unpleasant, chilly weather that there had been ever since we came into the place. Capt Grant and Mr. Sartwell were sitting below. The latter soon went out and, from having had some previous acquaintance here, he so managed as to obtain the refusal of a pretty good room, though in a very shabby house. We breakfasted with the same company that we had last spent the evening with, and several medical students besides, two of whom were Trask and Prescott. We conversed of a visit to Dr. Smith's laboratory that we had made the last night. This room is only two of the Collegiate rooms, converted into one by removing a partition. Seats are made, on one side of it, like those in the gallery of a church; and on the other, stands a large and long table, upon which the Doctor performs all his chemical experiments, and I suppose makes his dissections. In a closet adjoining were a few retorts, a Nooth's,[54] and a Woulfe's apparatus,[55] and a few other very common articles. One furnace, a number of students were then using, in the collection of phosphorus from calcined bones. None of them seemed to know much about the business, yet, by good luck, they had tolerably good success. Professor Siliman's apparatus for one lecture would have completely filled Doctor Smith's laboratory. From this subject we adverted to the College establishment in general; the want of rooms for the students, and the difficulty of obtaining them in the town. At last I alluded to the resolutions that Mr. Fish and I had come to in the morning. All hoped and believed that we should not be reduced to the necessity of returning to Connecticut; and Mr. Bush, our landlord, interested himself so much for us as to go to five or six places and intercede, in our behalf, though in vain. After breakfast a little, Doctor Smith called on us. We were, on the whole, sorry to see him, for we feared that when he learned we had given up the idea of living at Chandler's, he would think it was altogether owing to difficulty of our making, rather than his. We, however, stated to him the reasons of our procedures, and he was good enough to approve them. I finally concluded that on condition I might chose where I would eat, I would, rather than return home, give ten-dollars a quarter to Mr. Chandler for his room ready furnished. This, as things are in Hanover, was reasonable enough; and so the Doctor thought, and he went again to negotiate for us but all to no purpose, for on our terms, nothing short of twenty-five dollars would satisfy him. Doctor Smith once more took a circuit about town; but could induce none to entertain us.[56]

After dinner, Mr. Sartwell informed us that he had found a friend, destitute of a roommate, with whom he wished to study, but the owner of the chamber would not permit him to come in unless he would board in his family. As he supposed the man, however, would take any other gentleman, he proposed resigning the room, that he had obtained the refusal of in the morning, to Mr. Fish and me, on condition that one of us would board in the family and allow him to live where he was already engaged. As the boarding place was in Hanover unexceptionable, and as the room obtained was decent and on reasonable terms, we readily acceded to his proposals. Thus, was the apprehended necessity of being obliged to forego hearing a course of Doctor Smith's lectures, for which we had come so far, finally obviated. The remainder of the afternoon and evening we spent, pleasantly, with Mr. Atwater. He congratulated himself that, for the winter, he was still likely to enjoy the company of some of his Yale acquaintance; and we congratulated ourselves that we were, after so much vexation, tolerably accommodated.

Wednesday 28th.

With Mr. Sartwell, as conductor, Mr. Fish and I went after breakfast to view the chamber that we were calculating to obtain. The house in which it was stood probably a quarter of a mile from the College. It was a large, two-storied, gambrel roofed building, that had been left, externally, in such an unfinished state as to be, at this time, quite shabby. It was glazed only in but one or two rooms; and this had not been done till some individual had occasion to inhabit them. The whole house had, generally, since its erection been unoccupied; and in this situation, it was always said to be haunted. Groans, shakings of doors, and many other strange noises, had frequently terrified the weak and credulous in the neighbourhood; but, about fourteen months ago, there happened in the night such a disturbance in the garret that the assistance of the faculty of the College was called to suppress it. One unsuccessfull search was made for the occasioners of the alarm; but a second discovered several undergraduates in the very act. Making an example of these proved to be more efficacious in quieting the troubled spectres than half a dozen exorcisms, and the vicinage, afterwards, enjoyed undisturbed quiet, till, a short time since, two families took possession of all the lower part of the house. One front chamber, and one back one, had just been finished and were now engaged by medical students; the other front one wanted a hearth and windows to make it habitable. These were intended to be supplied in case any-body should appear to take the room. Mr. Fish and I made agreement for it and it was to be ready for our reception by Fryday at farthest. As the room was nicely enough finished, we now had a prospect of spending the winter, as it respected quarters, quite comfortably. But one thing was wanting, viz. an agreeable circle of acquaintances. This we were convinced we could not have from the town; and the students of the College were not yet assembled. A few of Doctor Smith's pupils were in town, but none, except Hartwell who boarded with him and perhaps Trask and Prescott, seemed at all congenial to our tastes. As I had hitherto been so much disappointed, I now determined not to expect too much of my fellow students that were to be; and I made up my mind to be, on the whole, contented with the society of Mr. Atwater, Mr. Francis, and Mr. Simmons. This latter gentleman was a student under Doctor Bacon, when I first went to Hartford. From our being both engaged in the same pursuits, we soon became acquainted; and to acquaintance there succeeded considerable intimacy. Mr. Simmons' education, preparatory to his entrance on professional studies, had been but little more than a common one; but from possessing excellent sense, a mind very susceptible of improvement, and withall a retentive memory, his stock of knowledge was considerable. His open and social disposition, joined to his mental acquirements, had heretofore pleased me, and I now imagined that I might, justly, anticipate much gratification from his company in Hanover. The year past he had spent in the place, and would probably likewise spend the year to come.

The remainder of this forenoon passed, as many others probably will, with Mr. Atwater. For the afternoon we planned a walk to Norwich, a town in Vermont, directly across the Connecticut. After dinner, accordingly, we set out upon our little excursion. We reached the river, after walking over just about a quarter of a mile of the pleasantest road I had seen since I reached the place. A good bridge, instead of a ferry, presented itself for our accommodation; but neither town, nor other signs of inhabitants, appeared on the Vermont side. After ascending a pretty steep hill, however, we had not only a view of a very handsome little village[57] at our feet; but Hanover appeared to much better advantage than I had ever seen it before. We lounged through the principal street, and were as much gratified at the sight of neat looking buildings, without broken windows, and of well cultivated grounds, as if we had never seen anything of the kind before.

38

After fatiguing ourselves pretty considerably, we returned home, supped, and in due time retired for the night.

Thursday 29th.

The early part of this day I devoted to books, though not to medical ones. I had opened that inexhaustible fund of wit and whim-wham, entitled Salmagundi, and was, for about the fortieth time I should think, so much entertained with it as not to think of closing it till near noon. After a morning of such inactivity, exercise of some kind seemed necessary; and walking, as being the most eligible, was pitched upon. The falls upon the Connecticut, about two miles below Hanover, I had not yet seen; and both Mr. Fish and Mr. Atwater were pleased with the idea of visiting them. About one o'clock, accordingly, we set out on this excursion without either knowing the way ourselves or obtaining any directions. Our route lay, generally, through bye paths, as the main road was perhaps three quarters of a mile from the river. We, however, guessed at the right course, and by three reached the spot we had been endeavouring to find. Here was presented to our view quite a considerable fall of water; trifling, to be sure, when compared with many others in the country; but such as did not fail of elevating my ideas and occasioning emotions of sublimity. The locks and canal that accommodated the navigation attracted my attention. I had never before had any adequate idea of their construction; and I therefore examined them with peculiar pleasure. In our return, we rambled out of all the direct paths, ascended every little eminence, and descended into every valley that appeared pleasant. Abundance of the ripe berries of the Gaultheria-Procumbens[58] caught our notice; and their aromatic taste induced us to delay considerable time in gathering them; so that we but just got home in season to take tea at our wanted time. Mr. Sartwell, I found waiting to release me, if I chose it, from my obligation to board in the family where he obtained his room, as another gentleman had offered himself to take my place. This was a very acceptable release; not because I expected to dislike my landlord or his fare, but because I should neither be with Mr.

Fish, Mr. Atwater, or anybody else of my acquaintance; and to go among strangers, with whom it was uncertain whether I should be pleased, I felt considerable reluctance; more especially as I was not to have the liberty of leaving them whenever I should think proper. Upon this I immediately applied to Mr. Atwater to speak a good word for me at Mr. Fuller's,[59] where he lived; and accordingly he did that very evening; and upon the strength of what he was pleased to say in my favour, I was admitted into the family. Mr. Fuller's place, with the grounds and fences pertaining to it, displays the most taste of any situation in Hanover. It is on the Norwich road; and is the nearest house, except one, to the bridge. Mr. Fuller was a native of Connecticut and a graduate of Yale-College; and hence his manners, and those of his family, together with their whole appearance, are totally different from anything around them. His whole family, at present, consists only of himself, one daughter and two or three servants. What ever induced him to settle in this place, or what his business may formerly have been, I am unable to say; but at present, he attends to nothing else but his boarding house. This he regulates so much after Connecticut fashions as to exclude almost every-body except Connecticutensians and those few graduates from Harvard and Yale that are occasionally under Dr. Smith's instruction. His fare is such as is to be found in the best boarding houses in New Haven and Hartford; and the same order and politeness is maintained as is to be found in every well-ordered family in any of our large towns. Nobody is admitted to his table who does not come well recommended, and thus, none but the best company is found at it.

This was the only place at which my class-mate Trumbull[60] would ever put up, when he used to visit Hanover; and it was the only place at which Mr. Atwater was willing to live on coming into the town.

Fryday–30th

Arose early, and dressed myself with uncommon alacrity, as this was the last time I expected to do it at Bush's. After washing etc. I called on Mr. Atwater, for the purpose of being introduced at

Mr. Fuller's. We went at the ringing of the College bell. At my first entrance into this mansion, I felt full conviction that it was not a whited sepulchre.[61] An air of the greatest neatness and regularity pervaded everything within; and I could easily see that all matters went smoothly and like clock-work. I was introduced to Miss Fuller, and was told that the master of the family was absent on a journey. Very soon, a couple of gentlemen entered, who were named to me as Mr. Thurston[62] and Mr. Putnam.[63] They were both Harvard graduates, and pupils of Doctor Smith. Mr. Thurston was tall, well built, and genteel, both in person and manners. His dress was elegant and of the latest fashion, but by no means indicating the fop. His face was good, though shewing evident marks of dissipation. Mr. Putnam was small and, at the present age, very engaging. His features were those of Professor Silliman in miniature; and at first glance I felt desirous of further acquaintance. These Harvardini, together with a Mr. Bradbury,[64] a man of much good sense, science, and real masculine beauty; and Mr. Woodbury,[65] a complete gentleman and scholar, both seniors in the College, for this morning made up our company. Our breakfast was served up with considerable elegance, and for a breakfast consisted of quite a variety of well dressed dishes. Such things as these, in Hanover, I was very far from expecting; and indeed I had but little reason to expect anything tolerable; for there were but about half a dozen houses, upon the Plain, as everybody calls it, into which I had not taken a peep; and none that I had seen promised much.

Conversation at table was not very brisk, owing, as I suppose, to our all being so much strangers to each other. Henry and I spent the forenoon in settling ourselves at our new room, which, from the circumstance of its being new, was far more cleanly and commodious than any apartments which we had yet seen, those at Mr. Fuller's excepted. The chamber directly across the entry from ours was occupied by Mr. Prescott, of whom I have heretofore spoken, and the one back of his, by a Mr. Hodges, neither of them very great bucks, but undoubtedly clever fellows.

At half after twelve, we took dinner. Our company had received the addition of a Mr. Brown[66] from Connecticut, a member of the senior class and a scholar. Mr. Atwater and I, on retiring, congratulated ourselves on having obtained admission to so excellent a circle.

The evening I devoted to Mr. Atwater. He is one of the most agreeable and instructive of companions; and I hope, most heartily, that our present intimacy will ripen into a lasting friendship.

Saturday 1st October.

Found myself, on first awaking, at my new lodgings, and congratulated myself upon it. The weather, as is usual in Hanover, gloomy and unpleasant. Hitherto, the sun has shone upon us only part of one day. I do not wonder at it, however, as Nature, here, wears her most horrid garb; and as if this were not sufficient, man seems to have exerted himself to the utmost to render her appearance more hideous. I concluded to indulge myself, to a late hour, this morning, as Mr. Atwater, Mr. Fish, and myself had resolved to begin the week with regular attendance at morning Prayers in the College Chapel; considering, that if there should be no higher motive for thus early rising, the promotion of health would be sufficient. A short walk with Mr. Atwater prepared us for breakfast, and the ringing of the College bell summoned us to the table.

Captain Dunham,[67] of Windsor, Vermont, had been invited to take a family meal with us. He is a man at least six-feet, four inches in height, and otherwise, proportionally large. His form is athletic; and every look, every motion, and every word he speaks, denote a large share both of the *vis corporis,* and *vis mentis* too. He was early educated at Dartmouth-College, but not choosing to follow either of the learned professions, he qualified himself for the army. He has, lately, held the commission of Captain at one of our western posts, but probably not receiving the promotion which he could not but be conscious of deserving, he has now laid it down; the discontent of his wife at such a situation being the ostensible reason. Attention to his property, of which considerable lies in and near Hanover, brought him hither upon the present occasion. At our breakfast table he, with propriety, took the lead in all the conversation; and his remarks were amusing, sensible, and judicious. Spent the forenoon in doing some writing that ought to have been done a week ago; and, from the disadvantage at which I laboured, felt most forcibly that procrastination is the thief of time. The afternoon passed, in a kind of hum-drum way, between Mr. Atwater and two or three persons that I cared nothing about, but, as they were to be fellow students, I felt myself under obligations to treat them with attention.

I learned that theological lectures are to be delivered, every Saturday, just before prayers, so attended accordingly; but as it was the first Saturday in the term, the lecture was dispensed with, and I found Doctor Wheelock[68] in the Desk instead of Professor Shurtliff.

This was the first time I had seen the old President, so I viewed him with a scrutinizing eye.

I was, at first glance, struck with his resemblance to a coarse wax figure of President Jefferson in Steward's Museum at Hartford. His nose, however, was much larger than that of the figure refered to; and it was shaped precisely like a spherical-triangle; and ergo, tho't I, as I made the comparison in my mind, the Doctor must be a great mathematician.

The Chapel is a small square building, from its situation, very much disfiguring a site, which from Nature has, in my view, no superfluous beauties. The outside of the building is two stories high, but low, and without windows in the upper part; though, in their stead, boards are painted in resemblance of sashes and Glass. The inside is arched, but in the centre is not higher than, perhaps, eighteen feet. The seats and aisles are narrow; and, as appears to me, injudiciously planned. In short, the whole interior precisely corresponds to my notions of subterraneous prisons and vaults, so often described in romance.

The President's Prayer did not correspond at all to my notions of supplication; for he seemed to be endeavouring to display his knowledge; and his phraseology was mere bombast. As prayers were attended rather earlier than usual, I concluded there was time for a walk; and accordingly I requested Mr. Fish & Mr.

Atwater to accompany me. Mr. Brown also, at our united solicitations, joined us; and as our Palinurus[69] conducted us across a field into a narrow path, which wound, very pleasantly, through a thick grove of large pine shrubs; and, at a considerable distance, opened into a handsome meadow on the bank of the Connecticut.

This evening the stage arrived from the southward; and Mr. Fish and I anxiously expected Francis, and our old friend Simmons, in it. I took care to be at the stage house in order to welcome them; but out of fourteen or fifteen passengers that allighted, there was not an individual that I knew. We concluded therefore, that they were coming on the beginning of the week in a private carriage; and so composed ourselves for the night.

Sabbath 2nd.

In consequence of our determination to attend prayers, I arose as soon as it was light and waited to hear the ringing of the bell. I found, however, that I was too far from the College for this; and saw that, on this account, regular attendance at Matins must be given up. I stepped into Mr. Prescott's room and learned that the hour of prayers had been some time past; so I proposed a walk, which was readily assented to. Mr. Prescott led me much such a route as Mr. Brown did last night. This morning, however, as we had more leisure, we descended to the meadow, and rambled about it some time, entertaining ourselves with conversation on several literary topics. Returning from breakfast, I met Mr. Francis, & I learned that he and Simmons arrived late last evening in a chaise. Simmons soon came along in company with Henry. We were, to be sure, most heartily glad to see these gentlemen; and we received them accordingly. Simmons is indeed a worthy fellow; and, in our circumstances, it was good for sore eyes to see him. I think I had not laughed so much, before, since I arrived at Hanover, as at this meeting. Before the bell rung for church, I called and spent a short time at Francis' room in the College, where I was introduced to several undergraduates whose names I do not now recollect. Thence I went to Mr. Simmon's room, in the chamber of Dr. Smith's office, where I was introduced to a Mr. Hildreth,[70] another Harvard graduate. This gentleman perhaps, at first view, might strike a stranger favourably; but from a slight scrutiny I thought I could discover, by nature, a little mind. I hope I am deceived in my notion, for I expect to frequent this room much.

Time for attendance on church drew nigh; but neither Mr. Fish, Mr. Atwater, nor myself knew where the seats appropriated to the medical students were. The last Sabbath, as there were so few people in the place, we did not think particularity of this kind necessary; but now the under-graduates were pretty generally here; and from our experience of collegiate customs, we supposed that in Hanover such an impropriety as placing ourselves among them, would be considered the unpardonable sin. In this dilemma we applied to Mr. Simmons, and after him to Mr. Francis; but neither of these gentlemen could attend the morning service. Mr. Francis, however, introduced us to a friend of his who very politely offered his service to wait on us to a seat, which we gratefully accepted. Professor Shurtliff was in the desk, and with a written sermon. I think it was considerably above medium; though by no means delivered in Doctor Dwight's eloquent and persuasive way.

Professor Shurtliff is undoubtedly a man of handsome talents and considerable science; but his parts are not brilliant. On examining the Triennial-Catalogue, I find that Parson Rich,[71] of the western parish of Say Brook, was his class-mate.

In the evening, after walking to and fro awhile in front of the College with Messrs Fish, Atwater, and Simmons, we went into the chapel at the tolling of the bell, and heard one of Doctor Wheelock's Sabbath-evening Prayers, commonly so much admired by the students.

To me, it appeared one of the greatest pieces of bombast I had ever heard, and unlike nothing so much as a humble supplication to the Throne of Grace. I believe it is certain that the faculty, and of course the students of this institution, have a relish for what would be called at Harvard, or Yale, or indeed in almost any part of the literary world, the turgid, the verbose, and the pompous. At any rate, I am confident that President Dwight would never have listened to such a frothy oration from any of his pupils as proceeded this evening from the lips of Doctor Wheelock.

About half after seven, Mr. Simmons called at our room; and a very pleasant chat we had till about nine. After his departure, I devoted a short time to my pen, and retired to rest.

Monday 3rd.

A dismal morning, as usual, in Hanover. I am, every day, more and more convinced that there is a moral fitness of one thing to another throughout the universe. Shivered with cold all the way to Mr. Fuller's; but an excellent cup of coffee, and a good breakfast otherwise, did much towards cheering me up.

I should know that the head of this family was either born or educated in Connecticut. I think the manners of Miss Fuller are far better than those of any lady in the place that I have yet seen; and I wish her person was less plain. According to the old observation however, beauty is but skin-deep. During the forenoon, the sun shone out so clearly that Mr. Atwater and I concluded we could not, willingly, spend the whole day at our rooms; but determined to make the most of what little fair weather Providence should be pleased to send us. As a pastime, however, till we should be ready to take our walk, I resorted to my pen, for Dr. Smith had not as yet begun his course of lectures, and till he should, we could not ascertain what would be his method. Desultory studies, to novices, we thought not very profitable. I was just seated when Mr. Prescott entered. He challenged me to vindicate the propriety, and utility, of making the dead-languages part of a liberal-education. This part of our collegiate-courses, I have been very frequently called upon to defend; and though it is, in reality, the very basis of all true erudition; yet to those who are not linguists, I find it as difficult to give correct notions upon the subject as of colours to a blind man, or sound to a deaf-one. Mr. Prescott was of opinion that the learned allow them to keep their places in our colleges and schools for the same reason that every man is allowed to burn his mouth with hot pudding. One has got caught, and he feels willing that another should be. We discoursed a long time, and Mr. Prescott could not help allowing that I had the advantage in the argument; for it was reasonable that none should decide who had not had experience, whether a knowledge of Latin, Greek, and Hebrew could be of service to himself; and he supposed a man who had the experience actualy would advocate the cause upon the principle just mentioned. He said, however, he had heard several batchelors of arts decry them. I enquired if this very conduct had not given him a contemptuous opinion of the knowledge and abilities of these same gentlemen in the languages; and whether such an inference would not be just, since so many men of the greatest reputation in the world had made a contrary declaration. He could not but answer in the affirmative; and he even conceded that one man of talents, not being able to turn them to a good account, would be no proof, that the greater number would not be benefited by them. This being granted, however, he could not see but that their opposers would be completely at the mercy of their advocates; and he could not discover how the truth was to be come at.

I thought we might rest pretty easy where we were; for the circumstance that so many learned men were educating their sons in this very course seemed to prove that the study of thc dead languages was not kept up upon the hot-pudding principle.

Parents, I thought, would never trick their children because they had been tricked, before them, especially in a manner so serious.

The example of France, who has made the rejection of languages a national act, was brought up. This argument, I thought, would go equally against the Christian religion, and the institution of the Sabbath. It could certainly not appear strange that men who were impolitic, ignorant, and silly enough to enact a law against these, should, like-wise, in the plenitude of their folly, close up the avenues of usefull knowledge. The writings of Thomas Paine[72] and Stephen Burroughs[73] upon this very point were mentioned. I replied that I should never think it worth my while to argue against the principles and sentiments of such men as these; and so, we parted. In the afternoon, I took the same route with Mr. Atwater that I had been, the preceding morning, with Mr. Prescott.

On arriving at the meadow, we continued our walk upon it. A narrow, but swift running stream, intercepted our progress. I boasted of my excellence in jumping, and reached but little more than half across it. I did not stop long in the water, however. Mr. A- declared himself clumsy, and jumped considerably over it.

After some time, we returned to our rooms, considerably fatigued; but after sitting a few moments, went to prayers, rather than break in upon a steady habit. The evening, Mr. A- insisted, I should spend in playing back-gammon with him; and I did accordingly.

Tuesday 4th.

This morning, Dr. Smith was to perform the operation for an aneurism, but at sixteen, or seventeen miles distance from Hanover. I felt desirous of seeing it; but to go so far for the purpose, would have been literally skinning a flint for three-pence, and spoiling a knife that cost six-pence. Had the patient, however, been within half a mile, I should have felt somewhat sheepish at attending, with such a concourse of students as the good Doctor commonly has with him.

The fact is, a student cannot be benefitted by practice, at any medical-college, unless he has the advantage of attending a hospital. The benefit that I propose to myself from spending this winter, and perhaps another, in this place will by no means result from seeing practice; but must be derived solely from the Anatomical Museum, the lectures, and the library.

Many of the medical students, in this instance, were unwise enough to be at much pains and expence to hire horses and to post off, break-fastless, to the patient's house, not to return, probably, till midnight, a dollar or two expended, a day's study lost, them selves fatigued, and six-cents worth gained. My books took up my attention, the chief of the day. At vespers, two dissertations were publicly read by two of the Senior-Class. I listened with open ears, but the readers spoke very low, were in one extreme of the chapel, and I in another, so that I could not hear enough to determine their topics. One thing was singular, the author of the last piece happened to have an inclination to attend a party of ladies, and so he was allowed to depute a friend to read his composition for him, as well as to take the benefit of the criticisms. Discipline, I think, must here be in his infancy, or second childhood, to allow such things.

Perhaps, however, getting an education by proxy is a modern Republican improvement. I trust it will never extend to Mother Yale. Doctor Wheelock in his observations, I thought, took rather strange ground; and I am inclined to think, if Doctor Dwight had been his opponent, he would have found it untenable.

I wonder how many times in the course of this Journal, I have made and shall make comparisons between Yale and her faculty and Dartmouth, and hers; and invariably to the disadvantage of the latter.

I suppose I should be thought prejudiced by people in general, though I am confident by few that are acquainted at both places. Mr. Hotchkiss, I remember says that sitting four years under Dwight and his Subs, invariably spoils a man for liking anybody else; and I believe the remark is partially true. I determined this evening to make strict enquiry, the first opportunity, into the course of studies pursued at Dartmouth, the characters of its instructors, and the laws and customs by which it is governed; and if I obtain satisfactory information, I resolve to note it down; and to place an account of Yale by its side. After tea I found I was like to be alone during the evening. My Cousin Dorrance at Middlebury came into my mind. I almost determined to take that place, in my way, as I returned home; but it was so long since I had either seen or heard from the person on whose account I was making these calculations, that I concluded to give Mr. Dorrance a line, and regulate my determinations according to the tenour of his answer.

The following letter I accordingly wrote and transmitted by the next mail.

Hanover 4th October 1808

Dear Sir,

So long a time has elapsed since you have seen, or, it is probable, heard from your Say-Brook friends and relations, that, very likely, many of them at present hold but a small place in your remembrance. Be that as it may, however, this letter will turn your attention to one who does not feel his regard for any individual, that he has once had affection for, lessen'd in the least by time and distance. The last four or five years of my life have been spent in such a manner as almost to preclude any intercourse between me and my old connexions, and I have, at present, but little more leisure; yet, as my pursuits have called me so far northward I cannot think of returning to my Father's without either hearing directly from or seeing you. I now expect to continue here, perhaps ten weeks longer; and I suppose it will not be a great deal out of my way to take Middlebury on my rout home. This I shall be happy to do if I can have the pleasure of meeting you, and becoming acquainted with your family. My parents and Mrs. Ely I left well a few weeks ago. They desired to join me in affectionate respect & regard to yourself and family, if I should trouble you with a letter. I shall expect a line from you in return, if you still make Middlebury your place of residence, and if not, this letter will probably join many of its fellows in Gideon Granger's office at Washington.

Permit me to assure you of my regard and remembrance—
W—T—

Mr. Joseph Dorrance. Middlebury

Wednesday 5th.

After breakfast Mr. Brown, the senior undergraduate, who I have before-mentioned as my fellow-boarder and acquaintance, accompanied me to my room. I now, for the first time, learned that he belonged to Brooklin, in Connecticut; and this, of course, made us much better companions.

We were soon interrupted, however, in our conversation by the entrance of Messrs Brewer, Sartwell, and a stranger, who was introduced by the name of Webber. Mr. Brewer is a gentleman who spent a short time last summer in Doctor Cogswell's office, and there I first made acquaintance with him.

He was rather dissatisfied at the little time which Dr. Cogswell was able to bestow upon his pupils, and learning that Mr. Fish and I were going to spend the winter in Hanover, he came to the same determination, and left Hartford immediately upon it. He had spent two years, previous to my knowledge of him, in the study of medicine, but was unlucky enough to pitch upon a mere puff-ball for his first instructor, and of course was much tinctured with the manners, habits, and notions of his master. The gentlemen retired in about half an hour.

At two o'clock I attended a public speaking in the College chapel. Four of the senior class declaimed and, according to law, ought to have spoken their own composition, but somehow that was dispensed with, for but one of the pieces was original. This was a Mr. Hartwell's, a gentleman who resembles John Chester 2nd of Wethersfield, Conn. in figure and general appearance, except in the particular that he has lost a leg. This misfortune, I should have supposed, would have been a sufficient excuse for his never mounting the rostrum, but he managed himself, very gracefully, on his crutch, and spoke with much propriety. His piece was on the advantages that have resulted to mankind from the invention of letters. The subject, in my opinion, was well treated, and as it was one which admitted ornament, his style was florid, though remote enough from the customary pomp of this place. The old Doctor who presided upon this occasion merely remarked upon the topic and was silent with regard to the speaker. Doctor Smith's first lecture was appointed at three o'clock this day, so I went from the chapel immediately to the laboratory. The Doctor did not make his appearance till some time after the whole medical-class was assembled, so that each individual had opportunity to make observations upon his fellows.

The majority of us were, undoubtedly, the wrong side of thirty, and a few, probably, over forty. I cannot say that I liked the general appearance over much. Such a motley colection I am sure I never set my eyes on before. Some seemed to be so awkwardly put together that, at first view, one would almost suppose that chance was the agent in their formation. The Clothes of some had, unquestionably, been in fashion as often as Hunks's Coat,[74] and they were, in general, so ludicrously put on that I hardly dared to trust myself with a second view. I found that I was like to be a pigmy in comparison with several and a giant with others. In order to view one from end to end, I found it necessary to bring my eyes into a perpendicular direction, like a squirrel. I enquired the name of this individual and found it was Abbot. The appearance and deportment of several denoted the complete gentleman, and among these were Thurston, Putnam, Hartwell (whom I saw at Doctor Smith's on first calling) and two or three that I did not know. On reviewing the company they did not appear half as bad as at first, and I perceived at last that much of my disgust arose from the total want of uniformity among them. I felt forcibly the propriety of establishing a uniform for all members of literary institutions, and I began to be conscious that much of the applause that the Students of Yale-College have gained for their appearance has been owing to a similarity of dress and behaviour, which they generally fall into by the end of the first term freshman-year.

Doctor Smith, after a while, slipped into the room and seated himself almost without our knowledge. I had really been expecting some of Professor Siliman's majesty and grace, and I felt a kind of disgust from my disappointment. His introductory address was altogether extemporaneous and couched in the most colloquial phrases. It was pithy, however, and in spite of its want of elegance, I could not but like it tolerably well. By this time I had got past being disappointed at anything that I should meet with in Hanover, and I made up my mind to be attentive to the matter only and not the manner of what my instructor and fellow students should say. As I had just got into this frame of mind, the embarassment of the Doctor's first address was over, and the man of true erudition, and the master of his profession, was manifest. He seemed determined that every one should have the full benefit of his instructions, however triflingly he had prepared himself to attend such a course. His subject was the Introduction to Chemistry. What he laid down was done with great precision, and his divisions were lucid and satisfactory.

Notwithstanding I felt myself as to any further disappointment completely callous, on leaving the lecture-room I could not help adverting to Professor Silliman.

This man, whom I have so often named, is a native of the western part of the State of Connecticut. At quite an early age, he was admitted to Yale-College, and passed through his pupilage with singular eclat.

He resided as a graduate in New Haven, after having the honours of the College, about three years; he now (being about 21) received the appointment of Tutor, the duties of which office, he discharged for five or six years to universal approbation. During this period he studied the profession of law, and was admitted to the Bar. Chemistry and Natural-History had always been favourite pursuits, and now, though he did not resign his Tutorship, he obtained leave of absence to prosecute these studies to better advantage in Philadelphia. Such were his attainments under Doctor Woodhouse, that it was said the students of the Pennsylvania-University viewed him much in the same light that they did the Doctor. At last, the Senatus-Academicus of Yale-College thought proper to offer him the Professorship of his favourite branches, which in due time he accepted, after spending a year or two at the University of Edinburgh and elsewhere in Europe. On his return to America, the liberality of Yale allowed him to build just such a laboratory as he thought proper. He accordingly improved, as is supposed, upon those of Europe, and took measures to have it furnished as liberally with apparatus as perhaps any in the world.

As a man, his talents are of the most popular kind. I know no person who possesses so much manly beauty as he, and his manners are the counterpart of his face and figure. To conclude all, he is a professing Christian, and in all human probability possesses a great share of genuine and unaffected piety.

Thursday 6th.

This the first day on which Doctor Smith is to deliver lectures regularly: a proper period, therefore, to make a distribution of my time. I breakfast at eight, and probably I shall not rise more than early enough to dress, wash, and put my room in order before this time. We shall not probably leave our boarding house before nine; at which time the lecture begins. This is to take our attention, invariably, till half past ten. From half past ten till noon I am to spend with my books; and from noon till one o'clock in exercises. At one I am called to dinner, where I shall probably be detained till towards two. At two, another lecture commences which lasts an hour and a half. The remainder of the afternoon to be devoted to study till tea time. The interval between supper and six o'clock, exercise again. From six till half after seven, a lecture; and the remainder of the evening, to my friends. Wednesday afternoons, on account of public speaking in the chapel, the lecture is not till three; and on account of the meeting of the two societies of the students in the evening there is to be none. There are to be only two lectures likewise on Saturdays.

For the remainder of the day, beside lecture time, I put my plan in execution and devoted myself to Chaptall's Chemistry.

In the evening I happened to be alone at my room. In the course of it Mr. Brown waited on me, as a Committee from one of the above mentioned literary-societies,[75] with a polite invitation to become a member. These institutions confine their favours, almost wholly, to the alumni of the College (and a selection only of them are admitted) and several literary characters who patronize them by becoming honourary members and giving all the other support in their power. Not more than one to a hundred of the medical students are, in general, requested to join them. They each possess a library of near a thousand volumes, which none but their members have the use of; and the compliment of membership, to those who are not Alumni of Dartmouth, consists in being allowed access to these books and that, too, free from the annual and necessary expences of the Society. This was a favour that I had no right to expect at all; but I thought it probable that from our belonging once to Yale it would be extended to us. I knew that the undergraduates here disliked the medical-students, in general, but I hoped we stood on better ground.

I returned thanks to Mr. Brown and promised him an answer the succeeding day.

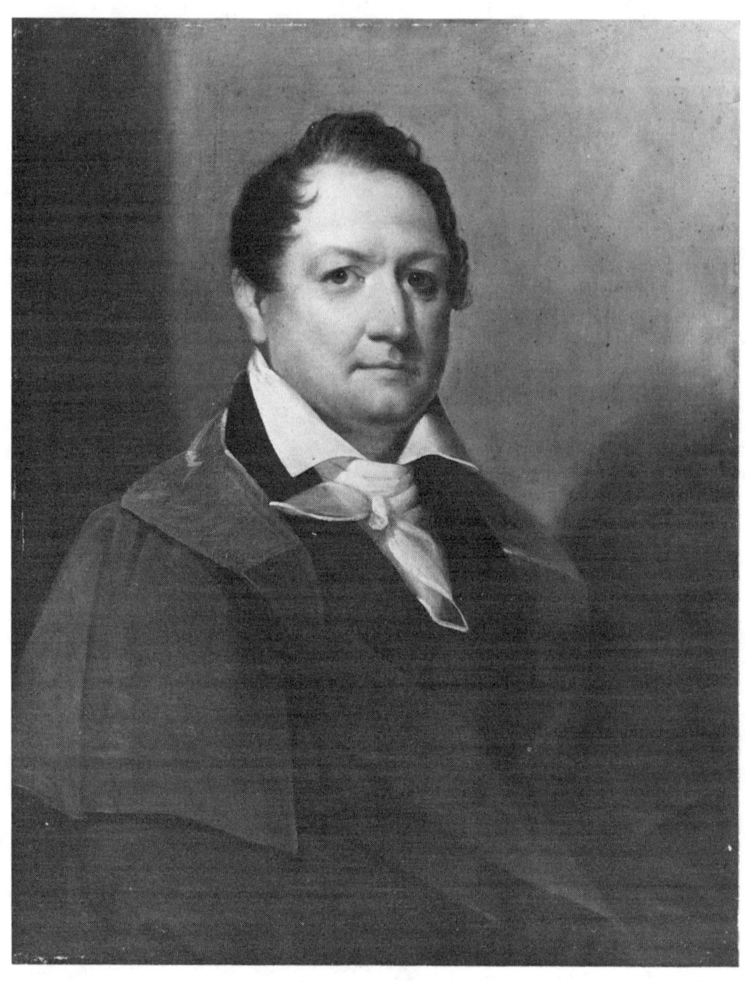

William Tully, Yale B.A. 1806, M.A. 1809, M.D. (Hon.) 1819. Professor of Materia Medica and Therapeutics 1829–1842. *Courtesy of the Yale University Art Gallery.*

JOURNAL

Hanover, N. H. Friday 7th October 1808

This day, both Mr. Fish and Mr. Atwater received an invitation to join the same society that had already paid me the compliment. We consulted together, and agreed to return our thanks to the *"Social-Friend's Society,"* for the favour done us, which we should most certainly be pleased to accept. In the course of the day, Mr. Brown was notified accordingly.

Our acquaintance Francis, whom I have before said was an undergraduate of the College, called on us in the evening. This gentleman belonged to the Society of the *"United Fraternity,"* the rival of the *"Social-Friends."* We knew that when any individuals came to the College, who it was thought would be a desirable acquisition to the societies, both calculated to give them an early and simultaneous invitation and stand an equal chance for gaining them.

From the circumstance of our coming from New Haven, we thought it probable that one society would dislike to have the other gain us; and we suspected that Francis on this principle intended to have got us into the *"United-Fraternity."* The event proved our conjectures true. Francis had, through mere laziness, procrastinated calling on us, and he relied upon our not being known sufficiently to be recommended to the other society. Dr. Smith had prevented our being strangers very long, and I, for my part, felt a little piqued that one who had known us a long time should shew us less attention, in our present circumstances, than those just made acquainted with us.

I took care, therefore, upon the present occasion to mention the politeness of the *"Social Friends,"* and our acceptance of their invitation. I intimated that my esteem of the society was much enhanced by the favour, as anything of the kind was unexpected.

Francis was mortified and vexed at his negligence, especially as he had now come as a Committee from his own society. He tried to persuade us to break our engagements (which he said was often done in similar cases) but we were immoveable, and kept on extrolling the *"Social Friends"* till, at last, he very coldly took leave, I do not care whether he forgets it, as long as we stay here.

—From Saturday 8th October to Wednesday 2nd November—

All this interval was passed in too monotonous a routine to be worth while to note the particular transactions of each day. I attended Dr. Smith's lectures regularly which were delivered uninteruptedly except for about three days when he was called to attend a sick brother in medicine, who had formerly administered to him, in similar circumstances, without fee or reward.

During this absence, Doctor Noyes[76] supplied Doctor Smith's place. This man had been some years a Tutor of the College and Assistant Lecturer to Smith. He is a man remarkable for his ingenuity and his mechanical talents, but like other great mechanists, he never finishes anything. I think, in the plain sailing of chemistry, he did as a lecturer quite as well as Doctor Smith. From having had an earlier education, he has more and better words at command than the good doctor; and from not being called to converse so much with the ignorant people of country places, his style was much less colloquial.

Of him I intend to speak further hereafter.

During this interval, our family at Mr. Fuller's was much enlarged. In addition to Thurston, Putnam, Bradbury, Woodbury, Brown, Atwater, and myself, there came a Mr. Martin,[77] a graduate from Brown University, who had already spent one year with Doctor Smith: A Mr. Johnson,[78] a young physician from the south-eastern part of New Hampshire, and two more of the senior-class of the College.

Martin was the exact counterpart of the Southerners of my class-mates; quite as foppish, quite as vain, and with just such superficial knowledge. Notwithstanding this, however, he was a pretty clever fellow. He had before been in the family.

Johnson possessed a great deal of wit, a great deal of life, vivacity, but was a notorious black-guard of those for whom he had conceived the least dislike. He was an excellent addition to our company, and invariably kept us in good humour and cheer. He could tell as entertaining a story, and sing as fine a song of any description as any person that I ever knew. With all his talents, both natural and acquired (& he had been graduated at Dartmouth and had heretofore spent two years under Doctor Smith), I believe he was a dissipated, unprincipled fellow. He had the faculty of being all things to all men, so of course accommodated himself, precisely, to our company, and only as our temporary companion, had we anything to do with him.

With regard to my society in general, Messrs Atwater, Fish and Simmons were the main point. Our table companions held the next rank, and after them, quite a small selection from the medical-class in general.

Though there was commonly a dislike between the undergraduates and medical students, yet as we were almost directly from New Haven we received much attention and civility from different members of the junior and senior-classes. In consideration of this, I felt a disposition to attend the College exercises in the chapel pretty punctually, and also morning and evening prayers, which was not required of the medical students. On the afternoon of—

Wednesday 2nd November.

Myself, Mr. Fish, Mr. Atwater, and Mr. Putnam were almost alone attending the Public Declamations. A dirty little scoundrel from the junior-class had parodied and altered into a very insulting piece against the medical students one of Peter Pindar's Blackguard Poems. He ascended the stage, turned himself towards, and directly addressed us. The language was too abusive and indecent to have been uttered in a brothel; and yet Doctor John Smith,[79] the Professor of Languages and an ordained clergyman, sat very composedly and listened to it. He even approved it when he had finished. I afterwards found that he looked to see who was present, when the speaker had begun, and discovering but one or two, beside Yalensians, he undoubtedly suffered him to proceed from a pique he had against Yale. We left the chapel mortified that our endeavours to please had not been thought worthy of more civil treatment. It was far from vexing us till we learned that the students boasted of having done a great feat; and that was beyond the endurance of us all.

We all agreed to indulge ourselves in some animadversions upon good manners in the form of an essay; one of us perhaps to publish in the Hanover Gazette, a newspaper issued from an office near the College. A short time, however, cooled down our wrath and there was but one essay written, and that was kept to ourselves. The following is a copy of it.

"Good Manners are the distinguishing Characteristics between the refined and the vulgar. On the scale which measures the politeness of a man is generally marked his real worth, and the estimation in which he is held. Good manners are of practical use in the business of life. They prevent asperities arising from a difference of views, and an opposition of sentiments. They always favour social intercourse, and they sometimes promote friendship between those whose principles are as opposite as the poles of the earth. By an attention to these little nicetices which mark the man of polished life, the Infidel Hayley and the Christian Conefer were enabled to mingle in each other's conversation with perfect cordiality. Hamilton and Burr could repair to the Jersey Shore and exchange shots without the least apparent interruption to good humour; and the ministers of the great contending nations in Europe can unite in social conviviality, and be on terms of perfect intimacy, either at the Court of St. James or the Cabinet of St. Cloud.

"There is an intimate connexion between manners and morals. In the Latin Language, one word denotes them both. In all human conduct an attentive observer will readily trace the effects of associated ideas. A man who has built a more elegant house than the one in which he has formerly lived, who has procured handsome furniture and a genteel dress, will, of course, acquire more refined sentiments and entertain better company.

"I have a thousand times marked the alteration which a clean

60

suit of clothes makes in the conduct of a school-boy; and often have I noticed in a coffee-house-throng the surprising stillness and regularity that has been produced merely by the company's laying aside their hats. No one ever puts on a Sabbath-day's dress without feeling somewhat starched; and though it be on a week day, the consequence is a more than ordinary circumspection of conduct.

"At all times we connect morality with decorum of behaviour in its possessor. The absence of the one invariably leads us to suspect the existence of the other. What opinion, for instance, should we form of the morality of him who should be guilty of obscenity in a polite assembly; or in the house of God should carry his child to receive the ordinance of Baptism in a Leathern-Apron.

"To one who duly estimates the advantages resulting from modes, and forms, from little attentions, and unexpensive ceremonies in improved society, an offence against civility will appear almost like the unpardonable sin; and in his view the perpetrator merits an equal punishment with him who impiously drew the veil from the Jewish sanctuary, or with those who had the unmannerly curiosity, and presumption, to look into the Tabernacle of the Lord before the horns of the Altar. The constantly abiding curse upon the posterity of Ham, was denounced in consequence of a breach of politeness. Misdemeanours, no less than crimes, have received the attention of wise Legislatures, in enacting Laws for the preservation of peace and good-order.

"What was said by a consummate judge of human-nature with respect to amusements, may, with great propriety, be applied to manners. Give me the direction of a people's manners and I care not who frames their laws. Arcadia was the most virtuous, because the most polished of the Grecian Territories. The illustrius Father of our Country, who was equally distinguished for the perfection of his tactics and for the polish of his manners, has shewn us the importance which the latter held, in his estimation, by the severity of his reproof to his Aid-de-Camp for wilfully bespattering with ink a mahogany-bureau; and by his repressing the unmannerly curiosity of one of his Generals by a most cutting reprimand. The General had received orders to march. He replied to the Commander in chief that he knew not his designs, nor whither he was going. Sir, said Washington, if I thought the Shirt on my back knew, I would burn it instantly.

"Politeness should always find a residence in a seminary of learning. The students of colleges are famed for the *adoration* which they pay to the *Muses*, and for credulity in believing themselves *inspired* by their influence. To *some*, however, the Delphic-Oracle is *dumb*; and their genius, like the Nihil-Album of the chemists, attaches itself to *productions not its own.* (Ghost of Pindar! forgive them, and blush not for the mutilation and prostitution of thy verse!) but were real politeness the shrine at which they would bow, her favour would be attainable by all, and her inspirations, unlike the *frantic effusions* of Sibbill or the unprofitable, vanity-puffing suggestions of the Nine, would confer an ornament of grace, and a crown of glory, upon the heads of her adorers.

"Viewing a collection of well-bred young men from the first families in the country, one would be ready to conclude them an unexceptionably polished and virtuous society were it not that sometimes an intruder, like Satan in the Garden of Eden with a perfect destitution of good-manners would, upon a public occasion, by a production manufactured out of the dregs from the sink, of the abomination of desolation, wound the ear of delicacy and induce his audience to lament that jackalls have lungs, and that toads are endued with the power to spit venom. But it would be the height of folly to take offense, either at the stupidity of a block or at the indecorous conduct of him whose soul is too small for a sense of propriety to reside in. Leave such a one, like Cain, to himself. It were better for him that a millstone were hanged about his neck and cast into the depth of the sea. Hush then, let no ebullition of my soul stir up the sediment of wrath or awaken my contempt, but come pity, weave a shroud for one that is dead, or at least beneath the notice of the living.

"The reputation of a college is much involved in the civility of its members. Should strangers at a public collegiate exercise be pointed out, and grossly insulted, by one to whom was assigned a part in the performances, the first impression would be that the good-breeding of the Students is to be suspected, and if suffered to proceed in his invective, the next would be that the Presiding-Professor is either tracing the radical of a Greek or Hebrew verb, or that an occasional ode, from Pindar's versification of the Devil's Book of Psalms, is calculated to assist the Sacrosancta-Theologia of the Doctor's Devotion; or certainly that he is ignorant of what the dignity of his station requires, and that the College is an Indian institution indeed."

Thursday 3rd.

This day, Mr. Atwater, Mr. Fish, Mr. Simmons, and myself formed a resolution to meet two evenings in a week for the purpose of examining each other upon the subjects of our lectures. My room was pitched upon as the place of rendezvous, because both Simmons and Atwater had room-mates, who we did not intend should join us.

Each of us, in rotation, was to be president of the meeting and examiner. We were occasionally to bring in some composition upon one or more of our subjects of pursuit; and the president of the evening and indeed the whole of us were to make the criticism.

From this little institution we propose much benefit. Our several instructors, hitherto, have been unable to attend to us as much in this way as we have wished; and we are of opinion that thorough examinations are even of more service than reviewing. As yet, we have had about five or six from Dr. Smith.

Tuesday and Friday evenings are to be the times of our meeting.

Fryday 4th.

Received another compliment, this day, from a Society.

It was from the Ὑπέρτατον-Βουλευτήριον or HIGH-COURT. This is rather a singular Institution. A few years ago, when some of the first graduates from any other College but Dartmouth began to attend Doctor Smith's School, they found a great dearth of such amusements as they had been accustomed to. This was owing to the dullness of Hanover, and the want of an eligible society. To obviate this, they met to-gether, a half-dozen perhaps in number, to make regulations to ensure their spending more time in each other's company. One evening an individual played a trick upon the rest for which they said he should receive trial; and immediately in a mock way they appointed, from their own number, a Chief-Justice, Assistant-Judges, an Advocate-General, a high Sherif—etc. Thus they went on, in imitation of the proceedings of a real court, allowed the criminal Counsel and Advocates, tried him, and, at last, sentenced him to forfeit a given quantity of wine for the benefit of the company.

This afforded them so much diversion that they agreed to become a standing Court, by the Greek denomination above mentioned, and to meet weekly. There would almost always be a cause or two to try every evening; one would be arraigned for riding out too much, another for not doing it enough; one for visiting the ladies too often, another for not doing it at all; one for studying too hard, another for doing nothing. The cause generally went in favour of him who had the best Counsel, or made the best argument himself; and which way-soever it turned, there was always either costs, or damages, that went for wine etc. for the use of the Society. Such a Bachanalian-Club at a college never wants supporters; and to tell the truth, all the good fellows, either among the medical-students or the Dartmouth graduates, belonged to it. The greater half of the medical-class, however, were excluded; and though they were not well bred enough to be gentlemen, yet they had sense enough to feel neglected. What aggravated this still more was that the High-Court students were the only ones whose company Doctor Smith kept out of the lecture room. He did not, to be sure, keep their company because they were members of this High-Court, but because their education had been such as made them agreeable to him, and because they were well-bred enough not to feel sheepish before him, on the one hand, or to treat him with too much freedom, on the other. Though the rest of the medical students did not live so as

64

to have a desire for Doctor Smith's visits, yet they could not bear to have anybody else do better; and so, it seems, they determined to raise a clamour, at some rate or other, and as they had no better handle for it, they cried out against such an institution as the High-Court's being allowed to exist in a college. The High Court very well knew that when they should be forced into the cognizance of Doctor Wheelock they could not be allowed to exist; as the tendency of their institution was really bad, though no ill effects had, at that time, resulted from it. Foreseeing their downfall, therefore, they publicly changed their society into one for medical examinations and exercises, and appointed occasional evenings for these purposes but yet, secretly, kept themselves just what they were formerly.

Thus they warded off the premeditated blow, but increased the hostility against themselves. This they cared nothing for, however. At this time they formed themselves a gold Medal to be worn by each member of the Society, having on one side, ϒΒ the initials of their name: below this the *Lancet*, the *Scalpel*, the *Trephine*, and the *amputating-knife*: at bottom *Sanitas*, and the individual's *name*. On the other side, at top was Υγεία, below were several *vials* of *Medicine*, and at bottom *Deo-Adjuvante*.

This further distinction was an eye-sore to their enemies, and caused almost open war between them.

This was their situation when I first got to Hanover. I had heard of their institution but troubled myself noth[ing] about it. The members I liked better than any other of my class mates, and had of course associated exclusively with them. They now gave me a very pressing invitation to become a member of their Court, a compliment that was not paid either Fish or Atwater. I gave them many thanks for their politeness, told them I feared I should make an unworthy member and that, on that account, I must decline the intended favour, though I should be highly gratified with their friendship and company as heretofore. My *real* reason for thus declining their invitation is too obvious to be mentioned.

Saturday 5th.

I understand that Professor Johny Smith thinks the Connecticut graduates ignorant of books, of men, and of manners. He says Yale College never goes deep into any thing and these remarks he made before his class. Oh! the jackass! I wonder what he thinks of the gentleman that spoke in public, the other day, the parody upon Pindar. He is, undoubtedly, a paragon of erudition and politeness. But our crime especially is neglect to pull off our hats as we passed him, and that before we knew him. May I never wear another hat if I lift mine from my head, ever, on his account. He is truly mighty tenacious of his dignity, and with good reason, for he has but very little to lose. I hardly know, however, why I spend words upon him, for all the students despise him. What a contrast between him and the good Dr. Nathan Smith, our Instructor in Medicine.

Tuesday 8th.

Doctor Ramsay has arrived, and I have this day had a view of him. He is a little rickety fellow, not four feet high, but with a face large enough, and a body big enough-round, for a man of 7 feet. The hump on his back is as large as a Pedlar's-Wallet, and his legs are semi-circles. He has a mighty commanding air, however, and his look seems to say, *"stand off, for I am holier than Thou."* Tomorrow evening, as a pompous advertisement in the Dartmouth Gazette says, he is to deliver "hints, on Medical Education at Rowley's Assembley-Hall." The ladies, and what not, are all invited. I hope none of them that calculate to attend are in a way of being like to "Tumble to pieces"; for if they are, I tremble for the consequences. I do not do right, however, to run on in this way, for Dr. Ramsay,[80] I suppose, is one of the first anatomists and physiologists in the world, though I am told a petulant disposition nearly spoils his usefullness. Dr. Smith will, undoubtedly, manage well enough with him, but most people think the wilderness of Fryburgh, [Maine], where he has actually pitched his tent, is the most proper place for him.

On Thursday his anatomical lectures commence; and next Sabbath evening he begins a course on natural-theology.

Thursday 10th.

I am convinced, from Ramsay's lecture last evening and that of to day, that the little man is an original. He has advanced a great many old ideas, but in a strange dress, and a great many as strange as the form in which they were presented. He seems determined to make all the ladies of Hanover Anatomists, as I infer from his observations of last night. I question very much whether he is like to have so much power over every Lady that sees him as he thinks he shall have. Why! his boasts seem to arrogate the talents of a Lovelace, and yet, I could not discover anything very captivating about him. It is best, perhaps, to suspend my judgement, for the present at least, though I can't well see the hazzard of advancing it now. I learn that he is to lecture morning and afternoon, and at that we shall hear Doctor Smith only once a day till Ramsay is through. I can't possibly find fault with the two specimens that we have had of this Edinburgh man, on the ground of his diction's being too colloquial. He is so full of his technics, his *non Pareils,* his *fauxpas,* and the like that, together with his Scotch dialect and accent which he sometimes uses, I question whether two thirds of his Class understand him fully.

For my part, I rejoice that I understand Latin and Greek and have a smattering of French, else I should be quite in the dark. I find advantage, too, from having read Burns' poems, for though I thought in the time of it that I was very near wasting my leisure, yet familiarity with the Scotch accent is now of service.

Saturday 12th.

Today the making out and printing of a catalogue[81] of the medical-class proposed. I was against it, for my part, because I did not want my name posted up in every tavern and blacksmith's shop in New-Hampshire and Massachusetts, along with such a set of fellows.

The High-Court to a man, I remarked, opposed it, I believe their motive was much the same as mine though they argued against it on the ground that it is going to be of no use, and that it will deceive the public; as it will purport that such and such individuals have attended this course of lectures, when it is well known that many expect to tarry but a part of it.

Those in favour of catalogues were the majority by one or two; but the opposers say their names shall not be used, for as we are not an incorporate body, the minority are not bound by the will of the majority. I suspect we shall have some difficulty about this matter, for Doctor Smith, I learn, is indifferent on the subject, and though it is a trifling one, yet these fellows set up in such an arbitrary way that they will use our names, whether we will or not, that I think it is best to see what can be done. I am sure one man has no right to make use of another's name without his permission.

Monday 14th.

We have succeded in getting Dr. Smith to prohibit the printing catalogues. He sees it will make a disturbance and, to keep peace, he has interfered. The catalogians say it is not Dr. Smith's business, and that they shall still go on. High times these, if a man's school sets itself above him! The Boulenterion to a man, together with us Connecticutensians, have been to every printer in the place and left our names with a prohibition of printing them. We shall send also to Haverhill and Windsor, the only two towns anywhere near that have printing offices.

Wednesday December 14th.

Quite a dearth of incident for a Journal for this some weeks past. The Lectures have gone on in their old round. Dr. Smith we admire and revere, more and more as we know him better.

Ramsay gives us information by his very extensive Anatomical-Museum and his lectures, but we have found he is a pettulant, conceited, ranting fellow. Dr. Smith is getting, by his assistance, the best set of anatomical-preparations in the country, and he says that Ramsay is helping him enough to earn his five hundred dollars a month, the wages which he receives. I have got acquainted with the Tutors of the College.

One I like much, and the other is by no means deficient in powers of mind, or scholarship, but he makes a fool of himself. I design to speak hereafter of all the officers of College, so shall say no more here.

At tea this evening Dr. Martin turned our attention to some elegiac lines in a Providence paper upon a very worthy and able friend of his—who was recently dead.

The elegy mentioned him under the fictitious name of Albert. Martin expatiated upon his benevolence, his kind-heartedness, his merit in general, and the respectability of his connexions. He remarked that he had married the only daughter of Judge Cushen. A class-mate rushed into my mind; I enquired and found, indeed, that it was Page—Page, one of the most profligate and vile fellows that disgraced my class. This fellow had visited the four quarters of the globe, but his talents which, to be sure, were great had only been corrupted by this extensive intercourse with mankind.

Whilst preparing for college in Middletown, Connecticut, he saw Miss Cushen, then a girl of sixteen and at a boarding school. After one or two interviews, he persuaded her to marry him privately, immediately after which, she happened to be sent for home without his seeing her again. Page continued his studies and at last joined College from which he was dismissed junior year.

After so long a time, without ever having had any intercourse with his wife after they parted at Middletown, he went to Judge Cushen, to whom he was totally unknown, and by way of introduction presented the Certificate of his Marriage.

His wife had never divulged the secret of her connexion, except to an old aunt that lived with her father, and she had been (for

two or three years, very unaccountably to her friends), refusing
the attentions of several of the first young men in the neighbourhood of Boston.

Page finally studied law and established himself in Providence.
This was the character that Martin had been extolling so highly.
I drew him on to say as much as he would (for I like to be a thorn
in the side of any man who has such notions) and then remarked
that he was my class-mate at Yale, and that I now remembered
hearing the circumstances of his marriage.

Martin, I believe, felt a little caught, and he hauled in his
horns somewhat by saying that he knew he had been rather dissipated.

Tuesday 20th.

To day several hundred catalogues made their appearance from
Middlebury, Vermont, with all our names upon them. I, for my
part, am most plaguey mad.

These musty old fellows think they shall acquire a vast deal of
fame by being posted up through the state as medical-students
at Dartmouth. I believe they think a catalogue with their names
upon it will be as good as a diploma of the degree of M.D.

Wednesday 21st.

Both Dr. Smith and Dr. Ramsay are vexed enough about these
catalogues. Ramsay has given the obtainers of them a confounded
scolding and I heartily rejoice at it.

We discover that Hildreth[82] has been the mainspring of the
business. The Boulenterion are determined to shew their spunk
upon the occasion, for they have appointed a committee of one,
and a resolute fellow he is too, to give Mr. Hildreth a kicking.

Monday 26th.

The Boulenterion Committee has done his duty. As his trust
was public. Mr. Hildreth took care to keep himself out of the
way for a long time, but at last Committee Whitman went to his

own room and kicked him out of it. Poor Hildreth has been so persecuted that I suppose he intends leaving the town, tomorrow or the day after.

May this be the fate of every one who conducts as he has.

I am this evening invited to attend the aniversary festival of the Boulenterion. They are to meet, on this occasion, in Rowley's Hall. I understand that a number of military-officers from Windsor are to be present. Mr. Fish and Mr. Atwater accompany me.

Two or three from the senior-class are invited.

Tuesday 27th.

Went, about six, to the High-Court. Mr. Thurston the committee to wait on us to the hall.

Found the court about to open.

Mr. Chief-Justice Hartwell[83] was at the head of a long table in quite an elevated chair: General-Advocate Dr. Woodbury,[84] at the upper part of one side and High Sheriff-Whitman,[85] placed opposite to him. Below Dr. Woodbury, on one side, were placed seats for the honourary members of the evening; and below Sheriff Whitman, on the other, were arranged the regular and standing members, all in uniform, with their hairs combed back and pretty plentifully powdered, and their medals suspended by a red ribbon from their necks. The High Sheriff opened the court very ceremoniously as well as pompously; Mr. Chief Justice informed us that this was only the second anniversary since the days of Hyppocrates [*sic*], but that it was now expected they would become much more frequent.

Mr. Thurston[86] pronounced an oration on Improvement in Medicine.

A song and tune were composed for the occasion by Dr. Alden,[87] and a poem was delivered by another member. The Chief-Justice closed these exercises with a most excellent address to those about to enter on the practice of medcine.

Another production had been expected from Dr. Putnam, but he unfortunately was at this time dangerously sick with an acute rheumatism.

The whole performances were good and entirely original.

The table was now at once spread by attendants with cold tongue, crackers, cake, cheese, with brandy and water.

When we had done with these, all were removed and glasses and wine were brought. A multitude of merry toasts were drank, a great variety of songs of every sort were sung, and that too extremely well by different persons in the company; and the evening was passed in social hilarity. Just about eleven o'clock the noise of a violin was heard in the house.

The chief-Justice ordered it to be called in and the table removed, and though we wanted the assistance of ladies, yet we contrived as it was to dance an hour or two.

Toward one we retired. There were, I think, about thirty of us; and I think our refreshments could not have cost the Boulenterion, less than as many dollars. This sum they had accumulated by their causes.

Wednesday 28th.

This morning quite a new disturbance broke out. The reproach thrown upon the catalogue party by the Boulenterions, and both Doctor Smith's and Doctor Ramsay's joining in it, and especially the festival of the last evening, had so disaffected the catalogians that they had said a great multitude of hard things both of Smith and their fellow students. A foolish fellow, one of the Tutors of the College, reported it to the Doctor, and that all his exertions for the good of the Class should meet with such a requital quite hurt his feelings. At the morning's lecture he spoke of what he had heard and animadverted pretty severely upon it. At last he left the room in tears. All felt the subject, and even these who had made the difficulty felt ashamed. The class was stopped from retiring; Mr. Atwater and myself were appointed a Committee to investigate the affair and set Dr. Smith at ease. Luckily, we were acquainted with the difficulty, and before any one had time to cool after the Dr.'s remarks, we carried the following paper round and every individual signed it.

"Supposing, from the remarks made to the medical-class by Dr. Smith that he must have been misinformed with respect to the feelings of his pupils, and wishing to remove an implication under which we labour, in consequence, as we believe of false and unmeaning reports, and which affects us, as a class, indiscriminately, we declare our entire satisfaction with the instruction and treatment in every respect that we have received; and that we have not, nor ever had, the least ground of complaint.." This paper we inclosed to Dr. Smith, with the following address:

"Dr. Smith's remarks, with regard to the disaffection of a considerable number of the class towards him, gave rise to an enquiry, which terminated in the appointment of a committee for the purpose of investigating the subject. After diligent enquiry, it appears that no such dissatisfaction does in reality exist, and that no single student has left, or intends to leave, the School on any such account; and consequently, that the information which Dr. Smith has received to this effect is wholly unfounded and false. The inclosed Declaration, as you will see, has been presented by the Committee of Investigation to every individual medical student, and by each signed with alacrity, as all were desirous of being cleared of the imputation of ingratitude for Dr. Smith's unwearied assiduity for the benefit of the Class."

I cannot say that I believe all this was literally true, but, as the matter was managed, nobody would own but that it was, and so we did right in stating it.

As the term now draws near to a close (there being but one day more to tarry), it may not be amiss to make some remarks upon the Institution, Faculty, and Government of Dartmouth College.

The Institution was founded about half a century ago by Dr. Eleazar-Wheelock, a clergiman from England, who came into this country with the benevolent intention of establishing a College for the Education and Christianization of the Aborigines.

Hanover was pitched upon, as being the most northerly settlement on the Connecticut. As few Indians could be persuaded to come to such a school, at first white people were admitted into it, though the funds were given for other purposes.

No great success attended the exertions in favour of the Indians, though, occasionally, one turned out well among them. The number of white students, however, was annually increasing till, at last, just before the founder's death, their number amounted to near one hundred.

Old Dr. Wheelock was an excellent man for his station; but unluckily he had reserved the right of nominating his successor, and at his death his son John was named. This man possessed a vast deal of book-knowledge and a very retentive memory, and these were his only qualifications. The students had hitherto been instructed by three men, called Professors, one of Languages, one of Philosophy, and one of Theology.

Upon the death of the first, the influence of the young President, with the Trustees, got a man appointed to fill the vacancy that was most miserably calculated for the place. This was no other than Doctor John Smith. The Trustees soon disliked him, but the office was given during life, or his pleasure, and their decree could not be recalled. As the other two professorships became vacant, however, young men, and men of a different stamp, were appointed. A Mr. Hubbard,[88] a really meritorious man, had that of Philosophy; and Mr. Shurtliff, that of Theology. They were neither of them very obsequious to the President, and one step led to another till he and Doctor Johny even refused to commune with them at the Sacrament Table.

The Professorship of Medicine and Chemistry, I have already given an ample account of.

Doctor Noyes was the first regular Tutor appointed by the Trustees. He was ingenious and learned, but so deficient in judgement as to allow his pupils to become his master. He officiated a year or two with no great applause, and resigned. A Mr. Brown succeeded him, a man of real excellence in his station; and Mr. Ayers,[89] an additional Tutor was appointed his colleague. Ayers is, in fact, not to multiply words, a dirty fellow.

In this state I found the College. Their principles of government are different from those at Yale.

At Dartmouth it is said that the students have come to years of discretion and if they do not do as they ought, the loss is their own. The Faculty decline using compulsion. Of advice they are liberal. A student may become an excellent scholar, but he is never obliged to study. There has never been any subordination either among the different classes of undergraduates, or among the officers and students.

Such a system as this cannot be very excellent; but yet it is far better than none. The example of the other New-England colleges, if nothing else, will, in time, lead to improvements; and in case it is ever removed from Hanover, it will undoubtedly be stationed in a place ten times more advantageously situated for a literary institution. Of Dr. Smith's School, which is connected with the College, I cannot speak too highly; but I have my doubts, whether after Dr. Smith any deserving man will take charge of it under so many inconveniences.

Thursday 29th.

This morning attended Doctor Smith's Valedictory Lecture.[90] The course was finished much sooner than I expected when I left home; but then I supposed I should hear perhaps but one lecture a day, whereas we have regularly had three. Hanover is so unpleasant that I, long ago, determined not to stay only till the winter term should be ended. The instructions for the remainder of the year, I understand, are three lectures and two examinations every week, a course of reading, and attendance upon all Dr. Smith's practice.

Degrees are confered at the annual commencements. The qualifications for that of Bachelor of Medicine are a liberal-education, with the degree of Bachelor of Arts; three years study of medicine; two courses of lectures on anatomy, physiology, hygeina, pathology, semiology, and therapeutics; passing an examination and submitting a dissertation to the acceptance of the Faculty of the College. Without a liberal education, the qualifications are the same, except that the term of study is extended to five years.

The following, as near as I can remember, are the heads of the Doctor's farewell instructions.

First he mentioned the importance of anatomy and physiology. He then spoke of the advantages that he had this winter given his class for attaining these branches, and remarked they were greater than he had in Edinburgh. He next dwelt upon the importance of chemistry. He said he had given us but a compendium of it, but he believed he had touched upon all its general principles. No lecturer can give every fact upon the subject. Something must remain to be got in private, from Books and otherwise. Every thing of importance, he said, in the experimenting line might be done with but little more than what is to be found in every private family. Chemistry, he said, was one of the eyes of medicine. It is also essential, to private gentlemen. A man, who does not understand the doctrine and laws of caloric, appears like an ass in everything.

This knowledge is essential to the explanation and true understanding of the most common and trivial phenomena of Nature. No physician but one who understands chemistry can possibly be aware of the influence of the air, heat, light, water, etc. upon his patient.

The Doctor said, however, that the subject of the benefits of chemistry was inexhaustible, and therefore he would not enter upon it. Botany is likewise of immense importance to the physician. The same may be said of natural history at large. Nobody can tell who has not experienced the benefit of a complete knowledge of the structure, functions, and uses, of the animal, vegetable, and mineral kingdoms. The Doctor next spoke of the immense sacrifices a good physician must make upon the altar of public good.

Indolence, ease, wealth, all, must be given up. The importance of physicians in society, the respect due to them, the necessity of their good behaviour, the indispensability of philosophy to medicine, etc., etc., were all ably touched upon. After this, he gave us considerable animadversion on observation and study.

When Dr. Smith closed, Cyrus Hartwell, in behalf and by the appointment of the class, read and presented an address to our good instructor. Our thanks were rendered for his great exertions.

The present state of medicine and surgery compared with what it was in New Hampshire before Dr. Smith's settlement among them. Our good wishes and prayers for Dr. Smith's long continuance. Valedictory.

The remainder of the forenoon I spent in taking a long walk with Atwater for the last time this winter in Hanover. In the beginning of the afternoon Mr. Fish and I packed up our things, and after that, received the farewell calls of most of our Friends.

Simmons and Hartwell promised to come and sit up with us till three in the morning, when we expected the Stage to leave the place. At tea I learned that Doctors Johnson and Webber were going to take the stage with us as far as Walpole. Mr. Atwater, on some account, was obliged to tarry till the ensuing Monday.

Mr. Brewer had long intended to be our companion.

The early part of the evening we spent in social chat. About ten we had a supper together at Mr. Fuller's, after which we played whist, and cribbage, ate fruit, and drank wine, till about one. As there were none but students going in the stage, we marched off after the driver, and persuaded him to start immediately. Hitherto, not a flake of snow had fallen, but now there was a violent storm. We went the first twenty miles to Windsor, however, on wheels, but by that time it had fallen to the depth of two feet. It was excessively cold, and had not the stories of Johnson and Webber, together with their songs, kept us in good humour, we should have suffered considerably.

As it was, we were generally pretty well chilled before we got to the end of each stage.

My sides, however, ached nearly as much with laughing at the merriment of Brothers Johnson and Webber as my feet with cold. We breakfasted at Windsor, were as antic as colts all the way to Walpole, where our company was reduced to Fish, Brewer, and myself.

On account of the depth of the snow, it was evening before we reached Bratleborough.

The next morning,

Saturday 31st.

We started at three, and reached Northampton to dinner. Brewer left us here. Fish and I got to Utley's in Suffield that night.

Sabbath, 1st January 1809.

In the morning, about eight o'clock, we were greeted by Mr. Fish's family at Hartford.

Monday 2nd.

Spent the day in visiting old friends; and on

Tuesday 3rd.

I embarked, about noon, in the Farmington-way-Stage, with but one passenger, and got to Nichols' at New Haven about eight in the evening. I called first at Mr. Bishop's, and found that both he and his wife were out of town, Mr. Baldwin's, Mr. Foster's, and Mr. Water's, were too far off to think of visiting in so short a time. I accordingly made, at once, for the College; called at Professor Silliman's Room, but did not find him; next at my classmate's, Tutor Strong's. He, also, was out.

Elisha Beebe Strong, at present a senior, was next thought of. He had gone out about half an hour ago. I now determined not to attempt finding anybody else but Clarke; and him, I had the good luck to catch at his room. After about half an hour's chat he called with me at the book-stores, where I made some purchases. He accompanied me to the stage-house and we parted.

The next morning . . . *Wednesday 4th* . . . I started for Say Brook, alone. We made such speed, however, that I reached my Father's at common breakfast-time.

Here ends my Journal; and glad enough of it am I. To tell the truth, this book might have contained some entertaining incidents; but I got so thoroughly satisfied with Journal-writing by the time Doctor Smith's lectures begun that I should have done no more about it had not I promised my friends some sketches of this kind.

This volume I have scribbled off at leisure hours from now and then a hint that I made, at a proper time, in my pocket-book;

but not half those hints have I noticed. I do not think I am a legitimate descendant of Job; so shall never undertake anything of this kind again.

End
of a Journal
to Hanover, a
residence there, and
a Return to Say Brook

SOURCES FOR THE NOTES

Bronson, Henry. Biographical Notice of Professor William Tully, M.D. *Proc. Conn. med. Soc.*, 1860, pp. 109–115; Reprinted in *Boston med. surg. J.*, 1861, *65*, 54–60.

Chase, Frederick. *History of Dartmouth College and the Town of Hanover, New Hampshire.* 2 vols. Vol. I, to 1815, Chase (Cambridge, 1891); Vol. II, 1815–1909, John King Lord (Concord, N.H., 1913).

Connecticut Valley Historical Society, *Papers and Proceedings, 1882–1903.* Vol. II. (Springfield, Mass., 1904). Tully in "The Early Physicians of Hampden County," pp. 170–174.

Dexter, F. B. *Biographical Sketches of Graduates of Yale College with Annals of the College History* (New York, 1885–1912). 6 vols.

Dictionary of American Biography. Edited by Allen Johnson and Dumas Malone (New York, 1928–1936). 20 vols.

Early Northampton. Published by the Betty Allen Chapter, Daughters of the American Revolution (Northampton, Mass., 1914).

Ferris, H. B. The Peregrinating Dr. William Tully, A.M., M.D. *Yale J. Biol. Med.*, 1932, *5*, 1–37.

Fulton, J. F. and Thomson, Elizabeth H. *Benjamin Silliman 1779–1864. Pathfinder in American Science.* (New York, 1947).

Hartford. First Church of Christ. *Commemorative Exercise . . . at its Two Hundred and Fiftieth Anniversary, October 11 and 12, 1883* (Hartford, Conn., 1883).

Kelly, H. A. and Burrage, W. L. *American Medical Biographies* (Baltimore, 1920).

Kingsley, W. L. *Yale College, a Sketch of its History* (New York, 1879). 2 vols. II, 74–76.

Lloyd Library of Botany, Pharmacy and Materia Medica Bulletin, No. 12, 1910, Pharmacy Series No. 2 (Cincinnati, Ohio). Tully, opp. p. 16.

Lord, J. K. See Chase, Frederick.

Love, W. DeL. *The Colonial History of Hartford Gathered from Original Sources* (Hartford, Conn., 1935).

Mead, Kate Campbell. William Tully of Connecticut, 1785–1859. *Johns Hopkins Hosp. Bull.*, 1916, *27*, 79–85.

New England Historical and Genealogical Register (Boston, 1849). Vol. III, 1849. The Tully family of Connecticut, p. 157.

FOOTNOTES

1. Dr. Mason Fitch Cogswell, B.A. Yale 1780. Studied medicine under his brother James Cogswell, an army surgeon. Practiced in Hartford, Connecticut 1789–1830, being famous for his skill in surgery and obstetrics. He was the first in the United States to ligate the common carotid artery for a tumor of the neck.

He was widely read, had one of the best libraries of his time, and was closely associated with the Hartford Wits, the important group of Revolutionary poets originally known as the Connecticut Wits. President of the Connecticut Medical Society for ten years, Cogswell played an important part in founding the Yale Medical Institution. He was offered the professorship of surgery and anatomy but urged the substitution of Dr. Nathan Smith of Dartmouth because he felt that Smith had the ability to make Yale's medical school the best in the country. Perhaps more important in his decision was his interest in the undeveloped field of education of the deaf and dumb. His own daughter Alice was thus handicapped by diphtheria(?) in infancy. Cogswell studied the teaching of the handicapped at Boston and later founded the Asylum for the Deaf and Dumb at Hartford. He also played an important role in founding the Retreat for the Insane in Hartford and the Connecticut General Hospital in New Haven. Tully studied under him in 1807 and 1809 and always considered him one of his closest friends.

2. Henry Fish (1788–1850) of Hartford, B.A. Yale 1806, M.B. Dartmouth 1810, M.D. Hon. Yale 1826. Practiced in New York City 1810–1819 and in Salisbury, Connecticut 1819–1845. (Dexter, VI, 27).

3. Thomas Bull, Jr., (1787–1850) of Hartford, B.A. Yale 1806, worked in his father's store 1806–1808 when he moved to the Western Reserve; insurance agent in New York City 1824–1850. (Dexter, VI, 11).

4. Amasa Loomis (1785–1824) of South Windsor, Connecticut, B.A. Yale 1807, ordained as minister of the Congregational Church in New Salem Society in Colchester, Connecticut 1813. (Dexter, IV, 141–152).

5. Judge Pierpont Edwards (1750–1826), B.A. College of New Jersey (Princeton) 1768, lawyer, politician, jurist, the eleventh and youngest child of the Rev. Jonathan Edwards. Practiced law in New Haven; military service in Connecticut during the Revolution. He had liberal views in politics, religion, and, if he is not belied, in morals as well. Championed liberalism and religious freedom against the dominant elements in Connecticut. For the last twenty years of his life was Judge of the District Court of Connecticut. (*D.A.B.*, VI, 43).

6. The Rev. Dr. Nathan Strong, B.A. Yale 1769.

7. "Canst thou by searching find out God? Canst thou find out the Almighty unto perfection?" Job 11, 7.

8. The Rev. Dr. Abel Flint, B.A. Yale 1785.

9. The new building of the First Church of Christ was completed at a cost of $32,014.26 and was dedicated on 3 December 1807. This house, like its

predecessors, was finished without artificial heat. Not until 1815 were stoves installed. (*Commemorative Exercises. . .* , pp. 161–163).

10. Daniel Wadsworth, Benjamin Silliman's brother-in-law, artist and architect. (Fulton and Thomson, *Benjamin Silliman*, p. 112).

11. "Young Tully . . . was then placed under the charge of the Rev. Frederick W. Hotchkiss, of his own parish, who instructed him, first in English studies, and afterwards in Latin and Greek, preparatory to college . . . 'an exceedingly defective preparation.' " (Bronson, Biographical Notice of Prof. William Tully, M.D., *Boston med. surg. J.*, 1861, *65*, 54–60).

12. A new building for the gaol was completed in the autumn of 1794. The prison occupied the lower part; in the upper stories there was a tavern known as "City Hall," whose main purpose, it was believed, was to give respectable people sent to prison for nonpayment of debts opportuntity for self-support while there. "It certainly attained that distinction and was never a popular social resort. . . ." (Love, pp. 291–292).

13. Nathan Strong (1748–1816) of Coventry, Yale 1769, classmate of Timothy Dwight, was invited to the ministry of this congregation 4 June 1773. Previously Tutor at Yale (1772–1773). John McCurdy Strong, son of Nathan Strong, drowned at East Hartford Ferry six days after graduation from Yale. (Dexter, VI, 63–64). Nathan Strong, Jr., was a graduate of Williams and Yale.

14. Jonathan Hubbard Sparhawk (1781–1819), M.B. Dartmouth 1802, M.D. 1812. Surgeon, United States Army and physician in Hartford, Connecticut.

15. He married Mary Potter of Enfield, Connecticut, "an excellent woman though a great sufferer from ill health." (Bronson, *Boston med. surg. J.*, 1862, *65*, 54–60).

16. Vermont. In this case probably means the Western Reserve.

17. Dr. Timothy Dwight (1752–1817), poet and clergyman, a grandson of Jonathan Edwards, and a leader of the Hartford Wits. President of Yale College 1795–1817. "Embraced the whole circle of human knowledge within his views; and gave every science its just estimation." (Silliman's oration at Dwight's funeral).

18. Elisha Beebe Strong (1788–1867) of Windsor, Connecticut, B.A. Yale 1809. Studied at Litchfield Law School, later at Canandaigua, New York. Member of New York State Assembly 1820, presiding judge of Monroe County, New York, Courts 1821–1823. (Dexter, VI, 281–282).

19. Dr. Oliver Wolcott (1760–1833), Republican Governor of Connecticut 1817. In 1783 he had satirized the Federalists in the state by resolving "That Government is one of those evils brought upon men by the fall, and ought always to be opposed by a free people; that we are free and determined never to be governed." (*Hartford Courant*, 5 August 1783).

20. Chief Justice Oliver Ellsworth (1745–1807), a prosperous Federalist farmer. When he retired from the court, he wrote a column "The Farmer's Repository" for the *Hartford Courant*, 1804–1805.

21. General Stephen Row Bradley (1754–1830), B.A. Yale 1776, LL.D., Hon. 1805. Became an aide-de-camp to General Wooster and served as a Commissary Major in the Revolution. Practiced law in Westminster, Vermont. In 1791 he went to the U.S. Senate as a Jeffersonian Republican; was a Senate leader and called the caucus which nominated Madison. Bradley disapproved of his war policy and retired from politics in 1813. Settled in Walpole, New Hampshire, across the Connecticut River from his old home. (Dexter, III, 549–552).

22. Justin Lyman appears to have deserved Tully's small opinion of him, for we have found no trace of him.

82

23. Jeremiah Atwater (1734–1811). Steward of the Yale College Commons 1778–1798.

24. Gideon Granger (1767–1822), born Suffield, Connecticut, Yale 1787. Admitted to the bar in 1789, and started to practice in Suffield. A mild liberal, he published articles in *American Mercury of Hartford* under the pseudonym of Algernon Sidney. Supported Jefferson who gave him important party responsibilities in Connecticut and appointed him Postmaster General 1801–1814. (*D.A.B.*, VII, 483).

25. The Pomeroy Tavern, which stood on the site of Draper's Hotel, was originally the homestead and inn of General Seth Pomeroy. Later his youngest son, Asahel, conducted it as a public house. . . . It became one of the most prominent buildings on Main Street. (*Early Northampton*, p. 111).

26. Dwight supported the majority of the congregation when Jonathan Edwards was dismissed from his pastorate for what would seem nowadays a minor disagreement on dogma.

27. Dr. Ebenezer Hunt, born about 1758.

28. Edmund Bliss (1786–1821), of Springfield, Massachusetts. B.A. Yale 1806; practiced law in Springfield. In College he was regarded by his classmates as eccentric, but gifted with a remarkable ability for argument. (Dexter, VI, 9).

29. Timothy Dwight's *Greenfield Hill*, 1794.

30. He probably derives this from the English abbreviation of *Hampshire*-Hants.

31. Political Observatory was a weekly newspaper published in Walpole from 1803–1809. Stanley Griswold (1763–1815), Yale 1786, was editor until 1805 when George W. Nichols succeeded him. In 1805 President Jefferson appointed Griswold his Secretary of Michigan Territory; in 1809 he was elected U.S. Senator from Ohio.

32. Charles Goldthwait Adams (1793–1856), B.A. Dartmouth 1810, entered Dartmouth Medical School in 1812 but did not graduate. M.A. Harvard 1816. Phi Beta Kappa. Practiced medicine in Keene, New Hampshire.

33. Bancroft Fowler (1775–1856), B.A. Yale 1796, studied law; Tutor at Williams College 1799–1800; Tutor at Yale 1800–1804; minister of the Congregational Church in Windsor, Connecticut, 1805–1819. (Dexter, V, 196–198).

34. Amos Dewey's Tavern at the northeast corner of the College Green, formerly owned by John Paine whose careless ways had been an ever-present thorn in the side of Eleazar Wheelock. (Chase, I, 264).

35. John Bush, B.A. Dartmouth 1789. Kept a boarding house in Hanover in early 1800's. Later taught school in Albany, New York.

36. Eleazer Hunt (1785?–1867), M.D. Hon. Yale 1826, entered Dartmouth Medical school in 1807 but did not graduate. He practiced in Coventry, Connecticut.

37. Abel Simmons (1885?–1818), M. B. Dartmouth 1810.

38. Josiah Prescott (1785–1864), M.B. Dartmouth 1810. Practiced in Belfast and Farmington, Maine.

39. Benjamin Trask (1785?–1831), M.B. Dartmouth 1815. Died in Montreal, Canada.

40. Roswell Shurtleff (1773–1861), B.A. Dartmouth 1799, D.D. University of Vermont 1834. Phi Beta Kappa. Philips Professor of Theology, Dartmouth, 1804–1827; Minister, College Chapel 1805–1827; Librarian 1810–1820.

41. William Atwater (1786–1833), B.A. Yale 1807. "A learned physician [of Westfield, Mass.], an interesting and witty companion. . . . His youngest son became a doctor." (Dexter, VI, 90).

42. *Salmagundi Papers*: a humorous periodical published in 1807–1808 by

Washington Irving, to which James K. Paulding and William Janice also contributed, satirizing life in New York; later issued as a book. Its purpose was "simply to instruct the young, reform the old, correct the town, and castigate the age." The *Dartmouth Gazette* carried one of the *Salmagundi* essays deriding the use of torpedoes to defend New York Harbor.

43. Dr. Alexander Ramsay (1754–1824), a Scotch anatomist. Previously Smith had taught the entire curriculum at Dartmouth Medical School except when Lyman Spalding (1775–1821), M.B. Harvard 1797, M.D. 1811; M.B. Dartmouth 1798, M.D. 1804, taught chemistry 1797–1798, and when Dr. Josiah Noyes, M.B. Dartmouth 1806, also taught chemistry 1807–1808. Ramsay came to the United States about 1800 and delivered a short course of lectures on anatomy and physiology in Columbia College. He later founded a school for anatomists in Fryeburg, Maine. A humpback, he has been called "the Calaban of Science."

44. Benjamin Silliman (1779–1864), "the father of American Scientific Education," B.A. Yale 1796, first Professor of Chemistry at Yale (1802–1853) at the age of 23. (Fulton and Thomson, *Benjamin Silliman*.)

45. This may have been Dr. Smith's first knowledge of plans he helped to bring to fruition in 1813.

46. Association of Yale with the Connecticut Medical Society was ended in 1884.

47. Harvard, after an excellent start in 1782, was having organizational troubles. In 1808 there were no graduates from Harvard Medical School. In 1809 and 1810 only two were given M.B. degrees each year.

48. Actually in Cornish, New Hampshire, on the opposite bank of the Connecticut River.

49. There is no other record of Smith ever attending Columbia.

50. Actually Dartmouth was the fourth (1797); the first school was founded at the College of Philadelphia (later University of Pennsylvania) in 1765; the second at King's College, New York (later Columbia), 1767; the third at Harvard in 1782.

51. William Chandler was Town Clerk in Hanover 1790–1793.

52. Thomas Sartwell of Walpole, New Hampshire, entered Dartmouth Medical School in 1807 but did not graduate.

53. Benjamin Smith Carnes entered Yale with the class of 1806 from Ashepoo, South Carolina. "He became dissipated, and died about 1810." (Dexter, VI, 15).

54. Dr. Nooth designed this glass apparatus for impregnating water with "fixed air," carbon dioxide, to prepare medicinal waters.

55. Woulfe's apparatus was a two-necked glass receptacle for preparation of gases by dropping a liquid onto a solid.

56. "Students shall board at no place disapproved by the President and no student shall in any case board at a tavern unless in the opinion of the executive authority of the College it is necessary on account of the scarcity of boarding houses or of the unreasonable price demanded for board by those who keep boarding houses or unless the Tavernkeeper be the parent or guardian of student and whoever violated this law and shall continue to board there after being reproved by the President shall thereafter cease to be considered and treated as a member of this College." *Minutes of the Annual Meeting of the Board of Trustees*, Dartmouth College, 1804.

57. Norwich, Vermont.

58. Wintergreen.

59. Caleb Fuller, B.A. Yale 1758. A deacon of Dartmouth College Church of Christ. Married in 1762 Hannah Weld of Attleboro, Massachusetts, whose father, the Rev. Habijah Weld, received his B.A. at Harvard, 1723.

60. Leverett Hubbard Trumbull (1788–1807) of Hartford, B.A. Yale 1806, the younger son of the Hon. John Trumbull (Yale 1767).

61. Matthew 23:27: "Woe unto you, scribes and Pharisees, hypocrites! for ye are like unto whited sepulchres, which indeed appear beautiful outward, but are within full of dead *men's* bones, and of all uncleanness."

62. John Thurston, B.A. Harvard 1807, M.D. Dartmouth 1818. Pupil of Nathan Smith. Died 1835.

63. James Putnam, B.A. Harvard 1808. Pupil of Nathan Smith. Died 1810.

64. William Bradbury (1783–1859), B.A. Dartmouth 1809. Phi Beta Kappa. Lawyer in Gloucester, Maine.

65. Levi Woodbury, born 1789 Francestown, New Hampshire. B.A. Dartmouth 1809, LL.D. 1823. Phi Beta Kappa. Judge, Supreme Court of New Hampshire; Governor 1823–1824. United States Senator 1825–1831. Secretary of the Navy 1831–1834.

66. Garrett G. Brown (1785–1870) of Bethlehem, Connecticut; B.A. Yale 1809. Studied at Andover Theological Seminary; licensed to preach 1811, but never held a charge; an itinerant teacher in South and Southwest. "Overpowering indolence was fatal to him." (Dexter, VI, 243).

67. Josiah Dunham (1769–1844), B.A. Dartmouth 1789. Phi Beta Kappa. M.A. Transylvania University 1823. Preceptor at Moor's School 1789–1793.

68. John Wheelock. "The first choice of President Wheelock [Eleazer], founder of Dartmouth College was his son Ralph, and his second choice was his stepson, the Rev. John Maltby, but the former was incapacitated by ill health and the latter died in 1771. The President, therefore named in his will as his successor his second son, John Wheelock, who at the death of his father (1795) was a young man of twenty-five, eight years out of college, and a Lieutenant Colonel in the Continental Army. He had no training, especially in divinity, then regarded as essential for the presidency of a college. . . ." (Lord, II, 1).

After a few years in office, "Dr. Wheelock was unfortunate in temper, and in a supreme self-sufficient obstinacy by which in his determination to have his own way at all hazards, he excited general hostility. He was fond of money, and careful about interest, which he often exacted at usurious rates, and by means not always irreproachable. Even his veracity was sometimes questioned. It will be readily inferred that he was not a favorite with his neighbors; even from his own brothers he was entirely estranged. Nor did he retain the love or respect of the students. He affected an involved, pedantic style of speech that exposed him to ridicule, and was sometimes ungrammatical and unintelligible." (Lord, II, 116).

69. The helmsman of Aeneas in Virgil's epic poem, the *Aeneid*.

70. Hosea Hildreth (1782–1835), B.A. Harvard 1805, M.A. Hon. Dartmouth 1817. Later a minister, he died in Sterling, Vermont.

71. Thomas Rich, M.A. Dartmouth 1799. Studied for the ministry, was ordained pastor of the Congregational Church, Saybrook, Connecticut, June 1804. Dismissed 5 September 1810.

72. Thomas Paine (1737–1809). His deism in *The Age of Reason* may have reminded Tully of the Epitaph quoted in the *Hanover Gazette* of 25 November 1809:

> "Reader, beneath this stone lies old Tom Paine
> Who living lied—now dead he *lies* again—
> Since Tom's no more, glance lightly o'er his merits.
> He's *sober* grown, altho' in midst of *spirits*.
> American Citizen.

85

73. Stephen Burroughs. Dartmouth's most notorious student was America's first celebrated confidence man. He shipped out as doctor on several merchantmen (without ever having studied medicine). Preached for four Sabbaths at Pelham for five dollars a Sabbath and was then hired to preach sixteen more. When suspected, he was given a Biblical verse as a text and told to compose a sermon on it. This he did to his congregation's entire satisfaction though he had previously been using his father's old sermons. This spoke well for his year and a quarter at Dartmouth, or for his native wit, or both.

For various misdeeds, including counterfeiting, he saw the inside of many of the jails in the United States and Canada. His memoirs were first published in Albany in 1811 and went through many editions, including an excellent one in 1924 from the Dial Press with a preface by his unabashed admirer, Robert Frost.

74. Hunk's coat. Hunk was a Pennsylvania Dutch expression, often of contempt. Usually used in reference to immigrants.

75. Social Friends was formed in 1783, possibly derived from the Linonian Society, then thirty years old at Yale. Early organized a library. The United Fraternity was organized in 1786 and at once voted to procure a library. Until 1825 both societies admitted medical students as well as undergraduates. Members of one society were not eligible for the other. In 1790 the books of both societies were brought together into a "Federal Library" open to all.

76. Dr. Josiah Noyes (1776–1853), B.A. Dartmouth 1801, M.A., M.B. 1806; M.D. elsewhere. Tutor 1807–1808 with Nathan Smith; later, 1809–1812, Professor of Chemistry and Pharmacy, College of Physicians and Surgeons, Fairfield, New York; Professor of Chemistry and Minerology, Hamilton, New York, 1812–1830.

77. John Russell Martin (1790–1817), B.A. Brown 1807, M.A., 1810; M.B. Dartmouth 1810.

78. Three Johnsons are listed in the Dartmouth Catalogue, Charles of Haverhill, Massachusetts, Oren of Plainfield, New Hampshire, and Abner of Bridgton, Maine. Presumably Oren is meant. He entered Dartmouth Medical School in 1806 but did not graduate.

79. Dr. John Smith, appointed pastor of the Church of Christ at Dartmouth College 25 November 1787 and Professor of Divinity in 1788, promptly became the focus of a church controversy which disturbed the college for years. He was considered to be overly influenced by President Wheelock. "He had many pleasant personal qualities, but he was not attractive as a preacher." (Lord, II, 16).

80. Letter from Dr. Nathan Smith to Dr. Lyman Spalding of Portsmouth, New Hampshire. Dartmouth College Library.

Dear Sir:

You may inform Mr. Taft that Dr. Ramsay is in my opinion the best Anatomist in the United States. I have seen his anatomical preparations, and have heard him lecture. You may also inform him, that Dr. Ramsay will not commence his Lectures till about the Tenth or Twelfth of Nov'r next, and if it should so happen that a number of students should apply after the lectures have advanced a few days, I will engage that they shall be repeated to them. The whole of my lectures on Surgery and Physic will be delivered after the 15th of Nov., so that should they come at the time you propose, they will have the benefit of the whole of our course, except Chemistry.

I wrote you before, that what I had undertaken this year would require the assistance of all my friends, and I must now make one more requisition on you. The plan we have chalked out to make me a complete Museum will require a number of subjects, therefore, I wish, if possible, that you would lay by a few for me. An infant with the placenta attached would be very agreeable. A child from six to ten or from ten to 15 would be very useful, or an adult subject, would not come amiss. If any of this kind of gentry can be obtained you can preserve them very easily by opening the cavities and immersing in new rum; just turn down the scalp and saw out a piece of the skull on one side, so as to admit the spirit, and so with the other cavities.

I will cheerfully pay you for any expense you may incur by the business. Perhaps you can engage Dr. Cutter and other physicians who would willingly oblige you and me to lend you some assistance.

If so that I could obtain those things, I would send to Portsmouth for that purpose. We shall want them through Nov. and Dec. and January, as we propose to drive a stroke of business in that line; and I am with sentiments of Esteem, and Respect your friend, etc.   NATHAN SMITH

81. The first printed catalogue of Dartmouth College, which contained a record of all prior graduates, was printed on one side of a large sheet—a broadside—and issued in 1786. Catalogues of the students in the Medical School were issued, also in broadside form, but in a small size, as early as 1806, when there was printed a "Catalogue of Medical Students and Students of College Who Attended Medical Lectures at Dartmouth College."

82. Hosea Hildreth. See note 70.

83. Cyrus Hartwell (1783–1816), B.A. Dartmouth 1806, M.B. 1809. Phi Beta Kappa. Died in Parsippany, New Jersey.

84. Levi Woodbury. See note 65.

85. Noah Whitman (1785–1854), B.A. Brown 1806, M.D. Dartmouth 1809. Practiced in Bridgewater, Massachusetts.

86. John Thurston. See note 62.

87. Ebenezer Alden (1788–1881), B.A. Harvard 1808, M.B. Dartmouth 1811, M.D. University of Pennsylvania 1812. Practiced in Randolph, Massachusetts. A trustee at Andover Theological Seminary and Amherst College.

88. John Hubbard (1759–1810), B.A. Dartmouth 1785, M.A. 1787. Phi Beta Kappa. Judge Probate, New Hampshire 1798–1802. Professor of Mathematics and Natural Philosophy 1804–1810.

89. Samuel Zyre (1786–1832), B.A. Dartmouth 1807, M.A., M.B. 1810. Phi Beta Kappa. M.D. University of Pennsylvania 1811. Preceptor, Moor's School 1807–1808. Tutor, Dartmouth College 1808–1810.

90. In 1806 one of Nathan Smith's students, William Ellsworth, recorded his valedictory to the graduating class:

VALEDICTORY CHARGE BY NATHAN SMITH

If the last sight of anything be attended with distressing emotions what must be the feelings of a teacher when he takes a last and farewell look at a number of his pupils, endeared to him by diligence in their studies by their most amiable deportment, and numerous instances of personal respect in his intercourse with them. Under the influence of these affections, I feel, Gentlemen, more than I am able to express, and were I permitted to obey the impulses of my heart, I would only squeeze your hands and by an affectionate silence convey to you my wishes for your future welfare. But as the custom of our University calls for a separation upon this public occasion, I shall endeavor to discharge this duty by briefly suggesting to you a few directions might be done, with but little more, than what is to be found, in every private family. Chemis-try, he said, was one of the eyes of Medicine. It is also essen-tial, to private Gentlemen — A man, who does not understand the doctrine, and Laws of balance, appears like an Ass. in everything. — This knowledge, is essential. to the explanation, and true understanding, of the most common, and trivial phenomena, of Nature. No Phy-sician, but one, who understands Chemistry, can possibly be aware, of the influence, of the air, heat, light, water, etc. upon his patient